Instructor's Guide for

PSYCHIATRIC/MENTAL HEALTH NURSING

Concepts of Care

Mary C. Townsend, RN, MN
Advanced Registered Nurse Practitioner
Clinical Nurse Specialist
Psychiatric/Mental Health Nursing

Nursing Consultant
Private Practice
Wichita, Kansas

Course Coordinator/Clinical Instructor
Psychiatric/Mental Health Nursing
El Dorado, Kansas

1993 F.A. Davis Company ● Philadelphia

CONTENTS

CHAPTER 1: AN INTRODUCTION TO THE CONCEPT OF STRESS

CHAPTER FOCUS

The focus of this chapter is to describe the concept of stress using various definitions that have been identified in the literature. The relationship between stress and illness is discussed.

LEARNING OBJECTIVES

After reading this chapter, the student will be able to:

1. Define *adaptation* and *maladaptation*.
2. Identify physiological responses to stress.
3. Explain the relationship between stress and "diseases of adaptation."
4. Describe the concept of stress as an environmental event.
5. Explain the concept of stress as a transaction between the individual and the environment.
6. Discuss adaptive coping strategies in the management of stress.

KEY TERMS

stress	fight or flight
adaptation	precipitating event
maladaptation	predisposing factors

CHAPTER OUTLINE/LECTURE NOTES

I. Introduction
    A. The word stress lacks a definitive definition.
    B. Adaptation as a healthy response to stress has been defined as restoration of homeostasis to the internal environmental system. This includes responses directed at stabilizing internal biological processes and psychological preservation of self-identity and self-esteem.
    C. Maladaptive responses are perceived as negative or unhealthy and occur when the integrity of the individual is disrupted.
II. Stress as a Biological Response
    A. This definition of stress is a result of research by Hans Selye. He defined stress as a "nonspecific response by the body to any stressor placed upon it." This syndrome of physical symptoms has come to be known as the "fight or flight syndrome."
    B. Selye called this general reaction of the body to stress the *general adaptation syndrome (GAS)*. He described the reaction in three distinct stages.
        1. Alarm reaction stage. During this stage, the physiological responses of the "fight or flight" syndrome are initiated.
        2. Stage of resistance. The individual uses the physiological responses of the first stage as a defense in the attempt to adapt to the stressor. If adaptation occurs, the third stage is prevented or delayed. Physiological symptoms may disappear.
        3. Stage of exhaustion. Occurs when there is a prolonged exposure to the stressor to which the body has become adjusted. The adaptive energy is depleted, and the individual can no longer draw from the resources for adaptation described in the first two stages. Disease of adaptation may occur, and without intervention for reversal, exhaustion and even death can ensue.
    C. The "Fight or Flight Syndrome"
        1. The initial stress response

       a. The hypothalamus stimulates the sympathetic nervous system, which in turn stimulates the adrenal medulla.

       b. The adrenal medulla releases epinephrine and norepinephrine into the bloodstream.

       c. Changes in the eye include pupil dilation and increased secretion from the lacrimal glands

       d. In the respiratory system, the bronchioles and pulmonary blood vessels are dilated and the respiration rate is increased.

       e. Changes in the cardiovascular system result in increases in force of contraction, cardiac output, heart rate, and blood pressure.

       f. The GI system undergoes decreases in motility and secretions. Sphincters are contracted.

       g. Effects on the liver result in increased glycogenolysis and gluconeogenesis and decreased glycogen synthesis.

       h. Ureter motility increases. In the bladder, the muscle itself contracts, while the sphincter relaxes.

       i. There is increased secretion from the sweat glands.

       j. The fat cells undergo lipolysis.

  2. The sustained stress response.

       a. The hypothalamus stimulates the pituitary gland.

       b. The pituitary gland releases ACTH, which stimulates the adrenal cortex.

          (1) The adrenal cortex releases glucocorticoids, resulting in increased gluconeogenesis, immunosuppression, and an anti-inflammatory response.

          (2) The adrenal cortex also releases mineralocorticoids, resulting in increased retention of sodium and water.

       c. The pituitary gland also releases vasopressin (ADH) which results in increases in blood pressure and fluid retention.

       d. The pituitary gland also releases growth hormone, which produces a direct effect on protein, carbohydrate and lipid metabolism, resulting in increased serum glucose and free fatty acids.

       e. The pituitary gland also releases hydrotropic hormone (TTH), which stimulates the thyroid gland resulting in an increase in the basal metabolic rate.

       f. The pituitary gland also releases gonadotropins, the initial response of which is an increase in secretion of sex hormones. Later, with sustained stress, secretion is suppressed, resulting in decreased libido or impotence.

III. Stress as an Environmental Event

  A. This concept defines stress as a "thing" or "event" that triggers the adaptive physiological and psychological responses in an individual. The event is one that creates change in the life pattern of the individual, requires significant adjustment in life style, and taxes available personal resources. The change can be either positive or negative.

  B. Easily measured by the Holmes and Rahe Social Readjustment Rating Scale.

  C. It is not known for certain whether stress overload merely predisposes a person to illness or actually precipitates it, but there does appear to be a clear, causal link.

  D. A weakness in the Holmes and Rahe tool is that it does not take into consideration the individual's personal perception of the event or their coping strategies and available support systems at the time of the life change.

IV. Stress as a Transaction between the Individual and the Environment

  A. This definition of stress emphasizes the *relationship* between the individual and the environment that is appraised by the individual as taxing or exceeding his or her resources and endangering his or her well-being.

  B. Precipitating event. A stimulus arising from the internal or external environment and is perceived by the individual in a specific manner.

  C. Individual's perception of the event. When an event occurs, an individual undergoes a primary appraisal and a secondary appraisal of the situation.

    1. Primary appraisal. The individual makes a judgment about the situation in one of the following ways.

       a. Irrelevant. When an event is judged irrelevant, the outcome holds no significance for the person.

       b. Benign-positive. This type of event is perceived as producing pleasure for the individual.

       c. Stress appraisal. These types of events include harm/loss, threat, and challenge.

          (1) Harm/loss. Refers to damage or loss already experienced by the individual.

          (2) Threatening. These types of events are perceived as anticipated harms or losses.

          (3) Challenges. With these types of events, the individual focuses on potential for gain or growth, rather than on risks associated with the event.

    2. Secondary appraisal. This type of appraisal is an assessment of skills, resources, and knowledge that the person possesses to deal with the situation.

3. The interaction between the primary appraisal of the event that has occurred and the secondary appraisal of available coping strategies determines the individual's quality of adaptation response to stress.
    D. Predisposing factors. Elements that influence how an individual perceives and responds to a stressful event. They include genetic influences, past experiences, and existing conditions.
        1. Genetic influences. Circumstances of an individual's life that are acquired by heredity (e.g., family history of physical and psychological conditions).
        2. Past experiences. Occurrences that result in learned patterns that can influence an individual's adaptation response (e.g., previous exposure to the stressor, learned coping responses, and degree of adaptation to previous stressors).
        3. Existing conditions. Vulnerabilities that influence the adequacy of the individual's physical, psychological, and social resources for dealing with adaptive demands (e.g., current health status, motivation, developmental maturity, severity and duration of the stressor, financial and educational resources, age, existing coping strategies, and a support system of caring others).
V.   Stress Management
    A. Stress management is the utilization of coping strategies in the response to stressful situations.
    B. Adaptive coping strategies protect the individual from harm and restore physical and psychological homeostasis.
    C. Coping strategies are considered maladaptive when the conflict being experienced goes unresolved, or intensifies.
    D. Some adaptive coping strategies include awareness, relaxation, meditation, interpersonal communication with caring other, problem solving, pets, music, and many others.
VII. Summary
VIII Review Questions

LEARNING ACTIVITIES

When the body encounters a stressor, it prepares itself for "fight or flight." Identify the adaptation responses that occur in the initial stress response in each of the physical components listed.

Physical component	Adaptation response
Adrenal Medulla	
Eye	
Respiratory System	
Cardiovascular System	
Gastrointestinal System	
Liver	
Urinary System	
Sweat Glands	
Fat Cells	

When the stress response is sustained for an extended period of time, the pituitary gland is stimulated by the hypothalamus to release a number of hormones. Match the ultimate physical effects listed below with the appropriate hormone that triggers the response.

_____ 1. Adrenocorticotropic hormone (ACTH)

_____ 2. Vasopressin (antidiuretic hormone [ADH])

_____ 3. Growth hormone

_____ 4. Thyrotropic hormone (TTH)

_____ 5. Gonadotropins

a. Results in increased serum glucose and free fatty acids.

b. Suppression of sex hormones resulting in decreased libido and impotence.

c. Increased gluconeogenesis; immunosuppression; anti-inflammatory response; increased sodium and water retention.

d. Increased basal metabolic rate.

e. Increased blood pressure (through constriction of blood vessels) and increased fluid retention.

List the value (in parentheses) for each event that you have experienced in the past 12 months in the column on the right. Add your total value to determine your risk of physical illness due to stress.

Holmes and Rahe Social Readjustment Rating Scale

Life Event	Value
Death of spouse (100)	_____
Divorce (73)	_____
Marital separation (65)	_____
Jail term (63)	_____
Death of close family member (63)	_____
Personal illness or injury (53)	_____
Marriage (50)	_____
Fired from work (47)	_____
Marital reconciliation (45)	_____
Retirement (45)	_____
Change in family member's health (44)	_____
Pregnancy (40)	_____
Sex difficulties (39)	_____
Addition to family (39)	_____
Business readjustment (39)	_____
Change in financial status (38)	_____
Death of close friend (37)	_____
Change to different line of work (36)	_____
Change in number of marital arguments (35)	_____
Mortgage or loan over $10,000 (31)	_____
Foreclosure of mortgage or loan (30)	_____
Change in work responsibilities (29)	_____
Son or daughter leaving home (29)	_____
Trouble with in-laws (29)	_____
Outstanding personal achievement (28)	_____
Spouse begins or stops work (26)	_____
Starting or finishing school (26)	_____
Change in living conditions (25)	_____
Revision of personal habits (24)	_____
Trouble with boss (23)	_____
Change in work hours, conditions (20)	_____
Change in residence (20)	_____
Change in schools (20)	_____
Change in recreational habits (19)	_____
Change in church activities (19)	_____
Change in social activities (18)	_____
Mortgage or loan under $10,000 (17)	_____
Change in sleeping habits (16)	_____
Change in number of family gatherings (15)	_____
Change in eating habits (15)	_____
Vacation (13)	_____
Christmas season (12)	_____
Minor violation of the law (11)	_____

Total Score   _____

Scoring: 0-150   No significant possibility of stress-related illness
            150-199   Mild Life Crisis level - 35% chance of illness
            200-299   Moderate Life Crisis level - 50% chance of illness
            300 or over Major Life Crisis level - 80% chance of illness

6

From the following case study, identify the predisposing factors (genetic influences, past experiences, and existing conditions) that influence Robert's adaptation response. What is the precipitating stressor in this situation?

Robert, age 56, was admitted to the emergency room of a large hospital at 2:00 a.m. after vomiting a large amount of blood. In doing the admitting assessment, the nurse learned the following about Robert:

His father and brother are both recovering alcoholics.

Robert had his first drink at age 12 and has been continually increasing the amount and frequency since that time.

His mother died of lung cancer when Robert was 23. She was a heavy smoker. Robert smokes 3 packages of cigarettes a day.

He has been hospitalized only once before, about 3 months ago, and diagnosed with an ulcer. The doctor told him at that time he must stop drinking and smoking in order for the ulcer to heal.

Robert is married and has three children. He has a long history of moving from one job to another, staying only until his drinking interferes with his work performance and attendance. He was fired from his job yesterday, and spent the evening and nighttime hours drinking two fifths of bourbon. He was engaged in this activity at the time the hematemesis began.

Because of the erratic job history, Robert and his wife experience severe financial difficulties. His wife shows much concern for Robert's condition and stays by his side during the emergency admission. She states to the nurse, "I want so much for our marriage to work, but he is drinking more and more all the time and still doesn't see his drinking as a problem. Every time he gets fired, he blames his boss."

STRESS AS A BIOLOGICAL RESPONSE

GENERAL ADAPTATION SYNDROME (GAS)

1. ALARM REACTION STAGE

2. STAGE OF RESISTANCE

3. STAGE OF EXHAUSTION

PERSONAL PERCEPTION
OF A STRESSFUL EVENT

PRIMARY APPRAISAL

    IRRELEVANT

    BENIGN-POSITIVE

    STRESSFUL

        HARM/LOSS

        THREAT

        CHALLENGE

SECONDARY APPRAISAL

    ASSESSMENT OF SKILLS, RESOURCES AND

    KNOWLEDGE TO DEAL WITH THE SITUATION.

PREDISPOSING FACTORS

GENETIC INFLUENCES

Family History of Physical and Psychological Conditions

Temperament

PAST EXPERIENCES

Learned Coping Patterns

Previous Exposure to Stress

EXISTING CONDITIONS

Vulnerabilities and Strengths that Influence Adaptation

(e.g., Health Status, Motivation, Developmental Maturity,

Financial and Educational Resources, and Support Systems)

CHAPTER 2: MENTAL HEALTH AND MENTAL ILLNESS

CHAPTER FOCUS

The focus of this chapter is to differentiate between mental health and mental illness. Various psychological responses to stress are explored, as well as cultural components that influence individual attitudes and behaviors toward mental illness.

LEARNING OBJECTIVES

After reading this chapter, the student will be able to:

1. Define *mental health* and *mental illness.*
2. Discuss cultural elements that influence attitudes toward mental health/mental illness.
3. Describe psychological adaptation responses to stress.
4. Identify correlation of adaptive/maladaptive behaviors to the mental health/mental illness continuum.

KEY TERMS

anxiety	psychosis
defense mechanisms	grief
compensation	anticipatory grief
denial	bereavement overload
displacement	rationalization
identification	reaction formation
intellectualization	regression
introjection	repression
isolation	sublimation
projection	suppression
neurosis	undoing

CHAPTER OUTLINE/LECTURE NOTES

I. Mental Health
    A. Defined as: "The successful adaptation to stressors from the internal or external environment, evidenced by thoughts, feelings, and behaviors that are age-appropriate and congruent with local and cultural norms."
II. Mental Illness
    A. Defined as: "Maladaptive responses to stressors from the internal or external environment, evidenced by thoughts, feelings, and behaviors that are incongruent with the local and cultural norms, and interfere with the individual's social, occupational, or physical functioning.
    B. Horwitz describes cultural influences that affect how individuals view mental illness. These include incomprehensibility (the inability of the general population to understand the motivation behind the behavior), and cultural relativity (the "normality" of behavior is determined by the culture).
III. Psychological Adaptation to Stress
    A. Anxiety and grief have been described as two major primary psychological response patterns to stress. A variety of thoughts, feelings, and behaviors are associated with each of these response patterns. Adaptation is determined by the degree to which the thoughts, feelings, and behaviors interfere with an individual's functioning.
    B. Anxiety
        1. Defined: A diffuse apprehension that is vague in nature and is associated with feelings of uncertainty

and helplessness.

2. Anxiety is extremely common in our society. Mild anxiety is adaptive and can provide motivation for survival.

3. Peplau identified four levels of anxiety.

   a. Mild: Seldom a problem. Associated with the tension of day-to-day living. Senses are sharp, motivation is increased, and awareness of the environment is heightened. Learning is enhanced.

   b. Moderate: Perceptual field diminishes. Less alert to environmental stimuli. Attention span and ability to concentrate decrease, although some learning can still occur. Muscular tension and restlessness may be evident.

   c. Severe: Perceptual field is so diminished that concentration centers on one detail only, or on many extraneous details. Very limited attention span. Physical symptoms may be evident. Virtually all behavior is aimed at relieving the anxiety.

   d. Panic: The most intense state. Individual is unable to focus on even one detail. Misperceptions of the environment are common, and there may be a loss of contact with reality. Behavior may be characterized by wild and desperate actions or by extreme withdrawal. Human function and communication with others is ineffective. Prolonged panic anxiety can lead to physical and emotional exhaustion, and can be a life-threatening situation.

4. Behavioral adaptation responses to anxiety

   a. At the mild level, individuals employ various coping mechanisms to deal with stress. A few of these include eating, drinking, sleeping, physical exercise, smoking, crying, laughing, and talking to someone with whom they feel comfortable.

   b. At the mild to moderate level, the ego calls upon defense mechanisms for protection, such as:

      (1) compensation - covering up a real or perceived weakness by emphasizing a trait one considers more desirable.

      (2) denial - refusal to acknowledge the existence of a real situation or the feelings associated with it.

      (3) displacement - feelings are transferred from one target to another that is considered less threatening or neutral.

      (4) identification - an attempt to increase self-worth by acquiring certain attributes and characteristics of an individual one admires.

      (5) intellectualization - an attempt to avoid expressing actual emotions associated with a stressful situation by using the intellectual processes of logic, reasoning, and analysis.

      (6) introjection - the beliefs and values of another individual are internalized and symbolically become a part of the self, to the extent that the feeling of separateness or distinctness is lost.

      (7) isolation - the separation of a thought or a memory from the feeling, tone, or emotions associated with it.

      (8) projection - feelings or impulses unacceptable to one's self are attributed to another person.

      (9) rationalization - attempting to make excuses or formulate logical reasons to justify unacceptable feelings or behaviors.

      (10) reaction formation - preventing unacceptable or undesirable thoughts or behaviors from being expressed by exaggerating opposite thoughts or types of behaviors.

      (11) regression - a retreat to an earlier level of development and the comfort measures associated with that level of functioning.

      (12) repression - the involuntary blocking of unpleasant feelings and experiences from one's awareness.

      (13) sublimation - the rechanneling of drives or impulses that are personally or socially unacceptable into activities that are more tolerable and constructive.

      (14) suppression - the voluntary blocking of unpleasant feelings and experiences from one's awareness.

      (15) undoing - a mechanism that is used to symbolically negate or cancel out a previous action or experience that one finds intolerable.

   c. Anxiety, at the moderate to severe level, that remains unresolved over an extended period of time can contribute to a number of physiological disorders. These may include, but are not limited to, tension and migraine headaches, bulimia nervosa, rheumatoid arthritis, ulcerative colitis, gastric and duodenal ulcers, asthma, irritable bowel syndrome, nausea and vomiting, gastritis, cardiac arrhythmias, premenstrual syndrome, muscle spasms, sexual dysfunction, and cancer. (Discussed at length in Chapter 25.)

d. Extended periods of repressed severe anxiety can result in psychoneurotic patterns of behaving. Neuroses are psychiatric disturbances, characterized by excessive anxiety or depression, disrupted bodily functions, unsatisfying interpersonal relationships, and behaviors that interfere with routine functioning. Examples of psychoneurotic disorders that are described in the DSM-III-R include anxiety disorders, somatoform disorders, and dissociative disorders. (Discussed at length in Chapters 20, 21, and 22.)

e. Extended periods of functioning at the panic level of anxiety may result in psychotic behavior. Psychoses are serious psychiatric disturbances characterized by the presence of delusions and/or hallucinations and the impairment of interpersonal functioning and relationship to the external world. Examples of psychotic responses to anxiety include the schizophrenic, schizoaffective, and delusional disorders. (Discussed at length in Chapter 18.)

B. Grief

1. Defined: The subjective state of emotional, physical and social responses to the loss of a valued entity. The loss may be real or perceived.

2. Kubler-Ross has identified 5 stages of the grief process through which individuals pass as a normal response to loss.

a. Denial - a stage of shock and disbelief.

b. Anger - anger felt for experiencing the loss is displaced upon the environment or turned inward on the self.

c. Bargaining - promises made to God for delaying the loss.

d. Depression - the full impact of the loss is felt. Disengagement from all association with the lost entity is initiated.

e. Acceptance - resignation that the loss has occurred. A feeling of peace regarding the loss is experienced.

3. Anticipatory grief. The experiencing of the grief process prior to the actual loss.

4. Resolution. Length of the grief process is entirely individual. It can last from a few weeks to years. It is influenced by a number of factors.

a. The experience of guilt for having had a "love-hate" relationship with the lost entity. Guilt often lengthens the grieving process.

b. Anticipatory grieving is thought to shorten the grief response when the loss actually occurs.

c. The length of the grief response is often extended when an individual has experienced a number of recent losses and when he or she is unable to complete one grieving process before another one begins.

d. Resolution of the grief response is thought to have occurred when an individual can look back on the relationship with the lost entity and accept both the pleasures and the disappointments (both the positive and negative aspects) of the association.

5. Maladaptive Grief Responses

a. Prolonged - intense preoccupation with memories of the lost entity for many years after the loss has occurred. Behavior is characterized by disorganization of functioning and intense emotional pain related to the lost entity.

b. Delayed/Inhibited - fixation in the denial stage of the grieving process. The loss is not experienced, but there may be evidence of psychophysiologic or psychoneurotic disorders.

c. Distorted - fixation in the anger stage of the grieving process. All the normal behaviors associated with grieving are exaggerated out of proportion to the situation. The individual turns the anger inward on the self and is consumed with overwhelming despair. Pathological depression is a distorted grief response. (Discussed in length in Chapter 19.)

IV. Mental Health/Mental Illness Continuum

A. In Figure 2-3, anxiety and grief are presented on a continuum according to degree of symptom severity. Disorders as they appear in the DSM-III-R are identified at their appropriate placement along the continuum.

V. The DSM-III-R Multiaxial Evaluation System

A. From the psychiatric diagnostic manual, individuals are evaluated on five axes.

1. Axis I - Clinical syndromes and V codes. Includes all mental disorders (except developmental disorders and personality disorders) and V codes (conditions that are not attributable to a mental disorder, but are a focus of attention or treatment).

2. Axis II - Developmental disorders and personality disorders.

3. Axis III - Physical disorders and conditions.

4. Axis IV - Severity of psychosocial stressors rated on a scale of 1 to 6 (none to catastrophic).

5. Axis V - Global assessment of functioning rated on the Global Assessment of Functioning (GAF) Scale that assesses mental health and mental illness.

VI. Summary

VII. Review Questions

LEARNING ACTIVITIES

On the following Mental Health/Mental Illness continuum, fill in the behavioral experiences or emotional disorders that correspond to the severity of anxiety or grief as it progresses along the continuum.

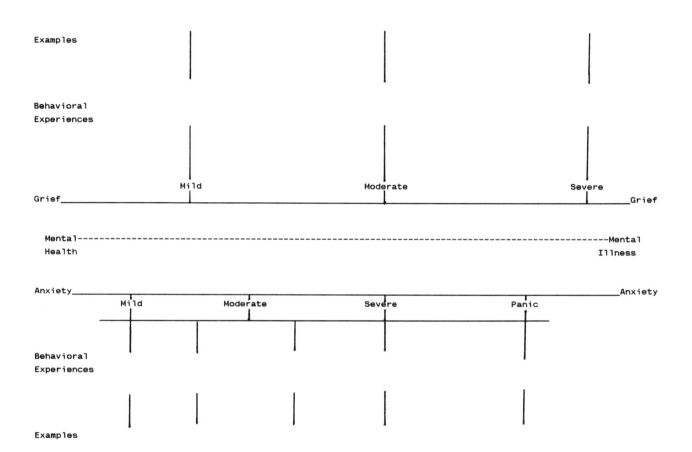

(An explanation of the solution for this activity may be found in Figure 2-3 of the text.)

EGO DEFENSE MECHANISMS - DEFINITIONS

In the box below, circle the names of the ego defense mechanisms defined as follows. The names may be identified in either direction vertically, horizontally, or diagonally. Number one is completed as an example.

1. Feelings are transferred from one target to another that is considered less threatening or neutral.
2. A mechanism that is used to symbolically negate or cancel out a previous action or experience that one finds intolerable.
3. The separation of a thought or a memory from the feeling tone or emotions associated with it.
4. Refusal to acknowledge the existence of a real situation or the feelings associated with it.
5. The beliefs and values of another individual are internalized and symbolically become a part of the self, to the extent that the feeling of separateness or distinctness is lost.
6. An attempt to increase self-worth by acquiring certain attributes and characteristics of an individual one admires.
7. A retreat to an earlier level of development and the comfort measures associated with that level of functioning.
8. Covering up a real or perceived weakness by emphasizing a trait one considers more desirable.
9. The involuntary blocking of unpleasant feelings and experiences from one's awareness.
10. Feelings or impulses unacceptable to one's self are attributed to another person.
11. The voluntary blocking of unpleasant feelings and experiences from one's awareness.
12. Attempting to make excuses or formulate logical reasons to justify unacceptable feelings or behaviors.

```
R A T I N T R O J E C T I O N
A L O M E N E N A T R N A M O
T B N A T I O N R O E B U S I
I U O N O T T U N I G A T N T
O S I U R A M I S S R N O R A
N N S N O I T A S N E P M O C
A O S D S E S N O M S R S T I
L I E O S T O I E R S O N I F
I R R I A R T C D E I J O N I
Z U P N R A A S T R O E A N T
A R P G L L U M I O N C I O N
T E U O P R O J N E I T I O E
I R S S U P R E S L A I N E D
O I I R E P R E S S I O N N I
N D I S P U C E M E N N T I O
```

16

THE GRIEF RESPONSE

Kubler-Ross identified five stages of the grief response: denial, anger, bargaining, depression and acceptance. Fill in the blank with the appropriate stage that describes the verbal or behavioral response. The first one is completed as an example.

1. "I never want to see you again!"   ___Anger___

2. "Cancer. It can't be! You must have made a mistake!"   _____

3. "At last I feel at peace with myself."   _____

4. "I'll go to church every Sunday if I can just live till my daughter grows up."   _____

5. "I wish I had been a better mother."   _____

6. "Why me? I don't deserve this!"   _____

7. "I'm feeling much better today. I think I should get a second opinion."   _____

8. "I feel as though I'm betraying my family. They depend on me so."   _____

9. "If God will only let me live till Christmas. I swear I won't ask for another thing."   _____

10. "My family is ready, and so I can rest easy now."   _____

CLINICAL EXERCISE

Have students keep a record of ego defense mechanisms they observe being used. These may be identified in the clinical setting, with their classmates, or with families and friends. Have them share these observations in their student group.

FOUR LEVELS OF ANXIETY

MILD ANXIETY: Increases motivation.
Sharpens the senses.
Learning is enhanced.

MODERATE ANXIETY: Perceptual field diminishes.
Attention span decreases.
Needs help with problem solving.

SEVERE ANXIETY: Can focus on one single detail.
Severely limited attention span.
Physical symptoms common.
Behavior aimed at relief of anxiety.

PANIC ANXIETY: Unable to focus on even one detail.
Misperception of environment is
common. May have delusions or
hallucinations.
Fear of dying or going insane.
Prolonged episode can lead to
physical or emotional
exhaustion.

EGO DEFENSE MECHANISMS

COMPENSATION

DENIAL

DISPLACEMENT

IDENTIFICATION

INTELLECTUALIZATION

INTROJECTION

ISOLATION

PROJECTION

RATIONALIZATION

REACTION FORMATION

REGRESSION

REPRESSION

SUBLIMATION

SUPPRESSION

UNDOING

GRIEF

FOUR STAGES (KUBLER-ROSS)

STAGE 1: DENIAL
- SHOCK AND DISBELIEF
- REFUSAL TO BELIEVE THE LOSS HAS OCCURRED

STAGE 2: ANGER
- ANGER FELT FOR EXPERIENCING THE LOSS IS DISPLACED UPON THE ENVIRONMENT OR TURNED INWARD ON THE SELF

STAGE 3: BARGAINING
- PROMISES MADE TO GOD FOR DELAYING THE LOSS

STAGE 4: DEPRESSION
- THE FULL IMPACT OF THE LOSS IS FELT
- DISENGAGEMENT FROM ALL ASSOCIATION WITH THE LOST ENTITY IS INITIATED

STAGE 5: ACCEPTANCE
- RESIGNATION THAT THE LOSS HAS OCCURRED
- A FEELING OF PEACE REGARDING THE LOSS IS EXPERIENCED

CHAPTER 3: THEORIES OF PERSONALITY DEVELOPMENT

CHAPTER FOCUS

The focus of this chapter is to provide background information for understanding the development of the personality. Major components of six leading theories are presented.

LEARNING OBJECTIVES

After reading this chapter, the student will be able to:

1. Define *personality.*
2. Identify the relevance of knowledge associated with personality development to nursing in the psychiatric/mental health setting.
3. Discuss the major components of the following developmental theories:
   a. Psychoanalytic Theory -- S. Freud
   b. Interpersonal Theory -- H.S. Sullivan
   c. Theory of Psychosocial Development -- E. Erikson
   d. Theory of Object Relations Development -- M. Mahler
   e. Cognitive Development Theory -- J. Piaget
   f. Theory of Moral Development -- L. Kohlberg

KEY TERMS

personality	superego
temperament	symbiotic
id	cognitive
ego	libido

CHAPTER OUTLINE/LECTURE NOTES

I. Introduction
   A. Personality is defined by the DSM-III-R as "deeply ingrained patterns of behavior, which include the way one relates to, perceives, and thinks about the environment and oneself."
   B. Life-cycle developmentalists believe that people continue to develop and change throughout life, thereby suggesting the possibility for renewal and growth in adults.
   C. Stages are identified by age. However, personality is influenced by temperament (inborn personality characteristics) and the environment.
   D. It is possible for behaviors from an unsuccessfully completed stage to be modified and corrected in a later stage.
   E. Stages overlap, and individuals may be working on tasks from more than one stage at a time.
   F. Individuals may become fixed in a certain stage and remain developmentally delayed.
   G. The DSM-III-R states that personality *disorders* occur when personality traits become inflexible and maladaptive, and cause their significant functional impairment or subjective distress.
II. Psychoanalytic Theory -- S. Freud
   A. Freud believed basic character was formed by five.
   B. He organized the structure of the personality into three major components.
      1. Id. Present at birth, the id serves to satisfy needs and achieve immediate gratification. It has been called the "pleasure principle."
      2. Ego. Begins to develop at age 4 to 6 months and works to maintain harmony between the external world,

the id, and the superego. Also called the "reality principle."
3. Superego. Development begins at about 3 to 6 years. It is comprised of the ego-ideal (the self-esteem that is developed in response to positive feedback) and the conscience (the culturally-influenced sense of right and wrong). May be referred to as the "perfection principle."

    C. Dynamics of the Personality
      1. Freud termed the force required for mental functioning *psychic energy*. It is transferred through all three components of the personality as the individual matures. If an excess of psychic energy is stored in one part of the personality, the behavior reflects that part of the personality.
      2. Freud termed the process by which the id invests energy into an object in an attempt to achieve gratification *cathexis*. Anticathexis is the use of psychic energy by the ego and the superego to control id impulses.
    D. Development of the Personality
      1. Freud identified five stages of development and the major developmental tasks of each.
        a. Oral stage (birth to 18 months). Relief from anxiety through oral gratification of needs.
        b. Anal stage (18 months to 3 years). Learning independence and control, with focus on the excretory function.
        c. Phallic stage (3 to 6 years). Identification with parent of same sex; development of sexual identity; focus is on genital organs.
        d. Latency stage (6 to 12 years). Sexuality is repressed; focus is on relationships with same-sex peers.
        e. Genital stage (13 to 20 years). Libido is reawakened as genital organs mature; focus is on relationships with members of the opposite sex.

III. Interpersonal Theory - H.S. Sullivan
    A. Based on the belief that individual behavior and personality development are the direct result of interpersonal relationships. The major components of this theory include:
      1. Anxiety. Viewed as a feeling of emotional discomfort, toward the relief or prevention of which all behavior is aimed.
      2. Satisfaction of needs. Fulfillment of all requirements associated with an individual's physiochemical environment.
      3. Interpersonal security. The feeling associated with relief from anxiety.
      4. Self-system. A collection of experiences, or security measures, adopted by the individual to protect against anxiety. Consists of three components:
        a. The "good me" - the part of the personality that develops in response to positive feedback.
        b. The "bad me" - the part of the personality that develops in response to negative feedback.
        c. The "not me" - the part of the personality that develops in response to situations that produce intense anxiety in the child.
    B. Stages of development
      1. Sullivan identified six developmental stages and the major tasks associated with each.
        a. Infancy (birth to 18 months). Relief from anxiety through oral gratification of needs.
        b. Childhood (18 months to 6 years). Learning to experience a delay in personal gratification without undo anxiety.
        c. Juvenile (6 to 9 years). Learning to form satisfactory peer relationships.
        d. Preadolescence (9 to 12 years). Learning to form satisfactory relationships with persons of same sex; the initiation of feelings of affection for another person.
        e. Early adolescence (12 to 14 years). Learning to form satisfactory relationships with persons of the opposite sex; developing a sense of identity.
        f. Late adolescence (14 to 21 years). Establishing self-identity; experiences satisfying relationships; working to develop a lasting, intimate opposite-sex relationship.

III. Theory of Psychosocial Development - E. Erikson
    A. Based on the influence of social processes on the development of the personality.
    B. Stages of development
      1. Erikson identified eight stages of development and the major tasks associated with each.
        a. Infancy (birth to 18 months). Trust vs. mistrust. To develop a trust in the mothering figure and be able to generalize it to others. Failure results in emotional dissatisfaction with self and others, suspiciousness, and difficulty with the interpersonal relationships.
        b. Early childhood (18 months to 3 years). Autonomy vs. shame and doubt. to gain some self-control and independence within the environment. Failure results in a lack of self-confidence, a lack of pride in the ability to perform, a sense of being controlled by others, and a rage against the self.

c. Late childhood (3 to 6 years). Initiative vs. guilt. To develop a sense of purpose and the ability to initiate and direct own activities. Failure results in feelings of inadequacy and guilt and the accepting of liability in situations for which he or she is not responsible.

d. School age (6 to 12 years). Industry vs. inferiority. To achieve a sense of self-confidence by learning, competing, performing successfully, and receiving recognition from significant others, peers, and acquaintances. Failure results in difficulty in interpersonal relationships due to feelings of inadequacy.

e. Adolescence (12 to 20 years). Identity vs. role confusion. To integrate the tasks mastered in the previous stages into a secure sense of self. Failure results in a sense of self-consciousness, doubt and confusion about one's role in life.

f. Young adulthood (20 to 30 years). Intimacy vs. isolation. To form an intense, lasting relationship or a commitment to another person, a cause, an institution, or a creative effort. Failure results in withdrawal, social isolation, aloneness, and the ability to form lasting, intimate relationships.

g. Adulthood (30 to 65 years). Generativity vs. stagnation. To achieve the life goals established for oneself, while also considering the welfare of future generations. Failure results in lack of concern for the welfare of others and total preoccupation with the self.

h. Old age (65 years to death). Ego integrity vs. despair. To review one's life and derive meaning from both positive and negative events, while achieving a positive sense of self-worth. Failure results in a sense of self-contempt and disgust with how life has progressed.

IV. Theory of Object Relations - M. Mahler

   A. Based on the separation-individuation process of the infant from the maternal figure (primary caregiver).

   B. Stages of development

      1. Mahler identified six phases and subphases through which the individual progresses on the way to object constancy. Major developmental tasks are also described.

         a. Phase I. Normal autism (birth to 1 month). Fulfillment of basic needs for survival and comfort. Fixation at this level can predispose to autistic disorder.

         b. Phase II. Symbiosis (1 to 5 months). Developing awareness of external source of need fulfillment. Lack of expected nurturing in this phase may lead to symbiotic psychosis.

         c. Phase III. Separation-individuation. The process of separating from mothering figure and the strengthening of the sense of self. Divided into four subphases.

            (1) Subphase 1. Differentiation. A primary recognition of separateness from the mother begins.

            (2) Subphase 2. Practicing. Increased independence through locomotor functioning; increased sense of separateness of self.

            (3) Subphase 3. Rapprochement. Acute awareness of separateness of self; learning to seek "emotional refueling" from mothering figure to maintain feeling of security.

            (4) Subphase 4. Consolidation. Sense of separateness established; on-the-way-to object constancy; able to internalize a sustained image of loved object/person when it is out of sight; resolution of separation anxiety.

V. Cognitive Development Theory - J. Piaget

   A. Based on the premise that human intelligence is an extension of biological adaptation, or one's ability for psychological adaptation to the environment.

   B. Stages of development

      1. Piaget identified four stages of development that are related to age, demonstrating at each successive stage a higher level of logical organization than at the previous stages. Major developmental tasks are also described.

         a. Sensorimotor (birth to 2 years). Within increased mobility and awareness develops a sense of self as separate from the external environment; the concept of object permanence emerges as the ability to form mental images evolves.

         b. Preoperational (2 to 6 years). Learning to express self with language; develops understanding of symbolic gestures; achievement of object permanence.

         c. Concrete operations (6 to 12 years). Learning to apply logic to thinking; develops understanding of reversibility and spatiality; learning to differentiate and classify; increased socialization and application of rules.

         d. Formal operations (12 to 15 + years). Learning to think and reason in abstract terms; makes and tests hypotheses; logical thinking and reasoning ability expand and are refined; cognitive maturity achieved.

VI. Theory of Moral Development - L. Kohlberg

   A. Stages of development

1. Not closely tied to specific age groups. More accurately determined by the individual's motivation behind the behavior.
2. Kohlberg identified three major levels of moral development, each of which is further subdivided into two stages each.
   a. Preconventional level (common from ages 4 to 10 years).
      (1) Punishment and obedience orientation. Behavior is motivated by fear of punishment.
      (2) Instrumental relativist orientation. Behavior is motivated by egocentrism and concern for self.
   b. Conventional level (common from ages 10 to 13 years and into adulthood).
      (1) Interpersonal concordance orientation. Behavior is motivated by the expectations of others; strong desire for approval and acceptance.
      (2) Law and order orientation. Behavior is motivated by respect for authority.
   c. Postconventional level (can occur from adolescence on).
      (1) Social contract legalistic orientation. Behavior is motivated by respect for universal laws and moral principles, and guided by an internal set of values.
      (2) Universal ethical principle orientation. Behavior is motivated by internalized principles of honor, justice, and respect for human dignity and guided by the conscience.

VII. Summary
VIII Review Questions

LEARNING ACTIVITIES

Identify whether each of the behaviors described below is being directed by the id, ego, or superego component of the personality. The first one is completed as an example.

___ID___ 1. Mary stole some make-up off the shelf at the department store.

_____ 2. Mary began to feel very guilty for taking the make-up after she got home with it.

_____ 3. Mary took the make-up back to the store and apologized to the clerk for taking it.

_____ 4. Two-year-old Sandy has a temper tantrum when her Mother takes the dangerous toy away from her.

_____ 5. Sandy sucks on her thumb for comfort.

_____ 6. Frankie wants to do well on the algebra test and stays home to study instead of going out with this friends.

_____ 7. Frankie does not do as well on the algebra test as he had hoped. He becomes despondent and refuses to come out of his room for days.

_____ 8. Jack joins his friends when they invite him to drink beer and smoke marijuana with them.

_____ 9. After having a few beers, Jack decides not to drive his car home.

_____ 10. Jack tells his parents he is sorry for drinking beer and smoking marijuana.

Match the behaviors or statements described on the right with Erikson's stages of development listed on the left. Both achievement and non-achievement are reflected in the choices. The first one is completed as an example.

__e__ 1. Trust

_____ 2. Mistrust

_____ 3. Autonomy

_____ 4. Shame and doubt

_____ 5. Initiative

_____ 6. Guilt

_____ 7. Industry

_____ 8. Inferiority

_____ 9. Identity

_____ 10. Role confusion

_____ 11. Intimacy

_____ 12. Isolation

_____ 13. Generativity

_____ 14. Stagnation

_____ 15. Ego integrity

_____ 16. Despair

a. "I don't like people. I'd rather be alone."

b. "Get away from me with that medicine. I know you are trying to poison me."

c. "I feel good about my life. I have a lot to be thankful for."

d. Five year old girl believes she is the cause of her parents' divorce.

e. "Sure, I'll loan you $10 till your next payday."

f. "I don't know what I want to do with my life. College? Work? What kind of job would I get anyway?"

g. "Mommy! Mommy! I made all A's on my report card!"

h. "I'll have to ask my husband. He's the decision-maker in our family."

i. "When I graduate from college I want to work with handicapped children."

j. "I plan to work as hard as necessary to help women achieve equality. I plan to see this happen before I die."

k. "I hate this place. No one cares what I do anyway. It's just a way to bring home a paycheck."

l. "Look, Mom! I ironed this blouse all by myself!"

m. "If only I could live my life over again. I'd do things so much differently. I feel like a nothing."

n. "I could never be a nurse. I'm not smart enough."

o. "Yes, I will be the chairperson for the cancer drive."

p. "I have been the Girl Scout leader for Troop 259 for 7 years now."

Match the statements/behaviors in the right hand column to the stages of moral development listed on the left.

_____ 1. Punishment and obedience orientation

a. "I really don't want to take care of this AIDS patient, but he needs care, and it is my moral and legal responsibility."

_____ 2. Instrumental relativist orientation

b. "I'll feed and water the pets because if I don't, I won't be allowed to go to the ballgame on Friday night."

_____ 3. Interpersonal concordance orientation

c. "I'll wear my seatbelt (even though it is uncomfortable and it wrinkles my dress) because it is the law."

_____ 4. Law and order orientation

d. "I'll tell him the truth about his prognosis because I would want to be told if it were me."

_____ 5. Social contract legalistic orientation

e. "I only drank the beer because everyone else was. They'd have thought I was a jerk if I didn't!"

_____ 6. Universal ethical principle orientation

f. "Okay, if you pay me $5.00 I won't tell Mom you skipped school."

STAGES OF DEVELOPMENT

Psychoanalytic Theory
(Sigmund Freud)

ORAL STAGE (BIRTH TO 18 MONTHS)

ANAL STAGE (18 MONTHS TO 3 YEARS)

PHALLIC STAGE (3 TO 6 YEARS)

LATENCY STAGE (6 TO 12 YEARS)

GENITAL STAGE (13 TO 20 YEARS)

STAGES OF DEVELOPMENT

Interpersonal Theory
(Harry Stack Sullivan)

INFANCY (BIRTH TO 18 MONTHS)

CHILDHOOD (18 MONTHS TO 6 YEARS)

JUVENILE (6 TO 9 YEARS)

PREADOLESCENCE (9 TO 12 YEARS)

EARLY ADOLESCENCE (12 TO 14 YEARS)

LATE ADOLESCENCE (14 TO 21 YEARS)

STAGES OF DEVELOPMENT

Psychosocial Therapy
(Erik Erikson)

TRUST vs. MISTRUST
Infancy (Birth to 18 Months)

AUTONOMY vs. SHAME AND DOUBT
Early Childhood (18 Months to 3 Years)

INITIATIVE vs. GUILT
Late Childhood (3 to 6 Years)

INDUSTRY vs. INFERIORITY
School Age (6 to 12 Years)

IDENTITY vs. ROLE CONFUSION
Adolescence (12 to 20 Years)

INTIMACY vs. ISOLATION
Young Adulthood (20 to 30 Years)

GENERATIVITY vs. STAGNATION
Adulthood (30 to 65 Years)

EGO INTEGRITY vs. DESPAIR
Old Age (65 Years to Death)

STAGES OF DEVELOPMENT

Theory of Object Relations
(Margaret Mahler)

I.   **NORMAL AUTISM (Birth to 1 Month)**

II.   **SYMBIOSIS (1 to 5 Months)**

III. **SEPARATION-INDIVIDUATION**

    A. **DIFFERENTIATION (5 to 10 Months)**

    B. **PRACTICING (10 to 16 Months)**

    C. **RAPPROCHEMENT (16 to 14 Months)**

    D. **CONSOLIDATION (24 to 36 Months)**

STAGES OF
COGNITIVE DEVELOPMENT

(Jean Piaget)

SENSORIMOTOR
(Birth to 2 Years)

PREOPERATIONAL
(2 to 6 Years)

CONCRETE OPERATIONS
(6 to 12 Years)

FORMAL OPERATIONS
(12 to 15+ Years)

STAGES OF MORAL DEVELOPMENT

(Lawrence Kohlberg)

I.   PRECONVENTIONAL (common from 4 to 10 years)

      A.   Punishment and Obedience Orientation

      B.   Instrumental Relativist Orientation

II.   CONVENTIONAL (common from 10 to 13 and into adulthood)

      A.   Interpersonal Concordance Orientation

      B.   Law and Order Orientation

III.   POSTCONVENTIONAL (can occur from adolescence on)

      A.   Social Contract Legalistic Orientation

      B.   Universal Ethical Principle Orientation

CHAPTER 4: RELATIONSHIP DEVELOPMENT

CHAPTER FOCUS

The focus of this chapter is to describe the role of the psychiatric nurse and the importance of a therapeutic relationship between patient and nurse. Steps in the development of a therapeutic relationship are discussed.

LEARNING OBJECTIVES

After reading this chapter, the student will be able to:

1. Describe the relevance of a therapeutic nurse-patient relationship.
2. Discuss the dynamics of a therapeutic nurse-patient relationship.
3. Discuss goals of the nurse-patient relationship.
4. Identify and discuss essential conditions for a therapeutic relationship to occur.
5. Describe the phases of relationship development and the tasks associated with each phase.

KEY TERMS

rapport
concrete thinking
confidentiality
unconditional positive regard

genuineness
empathy
sympathy

CHAPTER OUTLINE/LECTURE NOTES

I. Role of the Psychiatric Nurse
   A. Nursing has evolved through various roles as custodial caregiver and physician's handmaiden to being recognized as a unique, independent member of the professional health care team.
   B. Hildegard Peplau identified six subroles within the workrole of the nurse.
      1. Mother-surrogate: fulfills needs associated with mothering - basic needs, such as bathing, feeding, dressing, toileting, warning, disciplining, and approving.
      2. Technician: focus is on the competent, efficient, and correct performance of technical procedures.
      3. Manager: management and manipulation of the environment to improve conditions for patient recovery.
      4. Socializing agent: participation in social activities with the patient.
      5. Health teacher: identification of learning needs and provision of information required by the patient or family to improve the health situation.
      6. Counselor or psychotherapist: the use of "interpersonal techniques" to assist patients to learn to adapt to difficulties or changes in life experiences.
   C. Peplau believes the emphasis in psychiatric nursing is on the counseling or psychotherapeutic subrole.
   D. Peplau and Sullivan, both interpersonal therapists, emphasize the importance of relationship development in the provision of emotional care.
II. Dynamics of a Therapeutic Nurse-Patient Relationship
   A. Therapeutic nurse-patient relationship can only occur when each views the other as a unique human being. When this occurs, both participants have needs met by the relationship.
   B. Therapeutic relationships are goal oriented, and directed at learning and growth promotion.
   C. Goals are often achieved through use of the problem-solving model.
      1. Identify the patient's problem.
      2. Promote discussion of desired changes.
      3. Identify realistic changes.

4. Discuss aspects that cannot be realistically changed, and ways to more adaptively cope with them.
5. Discuss alternative strategies for creating changes patient desires to make.
6. Weigh benefits and consequences of each alternative.
7. Assist patient to select an alternative.
8. Encourage patient to implement the change.
9. Provide positive feedback for patient's attempts to create change.
10. Assist patient to evaluate outcomes of the change and make modifications as required.

III. Therapeutic Use of Self
A. Defined: The ability to use one's personality consciously and in full awareness in an attempt to establish relatedness and to structure nursing interventions.
B. Nurse must possess self-awareness, self-understanding, and a philosophical belief about life, death, and the overall human condition.

IV. Conditions Essential to Therapeutic Relationship Development
A. Rapport: implies special feelings on the part of both the patient and the nurse based on acceptance, warmth, friendliness, common interest, a sense of trust, and a non-judgmental attitude.
B. Trust: implies a feeling of confidence in another person's presence, reliability, integrity, veracity, and sincere desire to provide assistance when requested.
C. Respect: implies the dignity and worth of an individual regardless of his or her unacceptable behavior. Carl Rogers called this *unconditional positive* regard.
D. Genuineness: refers to the nurse's ability to be open, honest, and "real" in interactions with the patient. Genuineness implies congruence between what is felt and what is being expressed.
E. Empathy: a process wherein an individual is able to see beyond outward behavior, and sense accurately another's inner experience at a given point in time. With empathy, the nurse's feelings remain on an objective level. It differs from sympathy in that with sympathy the nurse actually shares what the patient is feeling, and experiences a need to alleviate distress.

V. Phases of Therapeutic Nurse-Patient Relationship
A. The Preinteraction Phase
1. Obtain information about the patient from chart, significant others, or other health team members.
2. Examine one's own feelings, fears, and anxieties about working with a particular patient.
B. The Orientation (Introductory) Phase
1. Create environment of trust and rapport.
2. Establish contract for intervention.
3. Gather assessment data.
4. Identify patient's strengths and weaknesses.
5. Formulate nursing diagnoses.
6. Set mutually agreeable goals.
7. Develop a realistic plan of action.
8. Explore feelings of both patient and nurse.
C. The Working Phase
1. Maintain trust and rapport.
2. Promote patient's insight and perception of reality.
3. Use problem-solving model to work toward achievement of established goals.
4. Overcome resistance behaviors.
5. Continuously evaluate progress toward goal attainment.
D. Termination Phase
1. Therapeutic conclusion of the relationship occurs when:
a. Progress has been made toward attainment of the goals.
b. A plan of action for more adaptive coping with future stressful situations has been established
c. Feelings about termination of the relationship are recognized and explored.

VI. Summary
VII. Review Questions

LEARNING ACTIVITIES

Situation: Pam comes to the psychiatric clinic for assistance with more adaptive coping. Nurse Jones will be her therapist.

Match the behaviors described on the right with the essential condition for therapeutic relationship development listed on the left.

_____ 1. Rapport

_____ 2. Trust

_____ 3. Respect

_____ 4. Genuineness

_____ 5. Empathy

a. Nurse Jones does not approve of Pam's gay lifestyle, but accepts her unconditionally nonetheless.

b. Nurse Jones and Pam develop an immediate mutual regard for each other.

c. Pam knows that Nurse Jones is always honest with her and will tell her the truth even if it is sometimes painful.

d. Pam knows that Nurse Jones will not tell anyone else about what they discuss in therapy.

e. When Pam talks about her problems, Nurse Jones listens objectively and encourages Pam to reflect on her feelings about the situation.

PHASES OF RELATIONSHIP DEVELOPMENT

Identify the appropriate phase of relationship development for each of the following tasks. The four phases include:

a.   Preinteraction Phase
b.   Orientation (Introductory) Phase
c.   Working Phase
d.   Termination Phase

The first one is completed as an example.

___b___   1. Pam and Nurse Jones set goals for their time together.

_____   2. Nurse Jones reads Pam's previous medical records.

_____   3. Having identified Pam's problem, they discuss aspects for possible change and ways to accomplish it.

_____   4. They establish a mutual contract for intervention.

_____   5. The established goals have been met.

_____   6. Nurse Jones explores her feelings about working with a gay person.

_____   7. Pam weighs the benefits and consequences of various alternatives for change.

_____   8. Pam and Nurse Jones discuss a plan of action for Pam to employ in the advent of stressful situations following therapy.

_____   9. Pam cries and says she cannot stop coming to therapy.

_____   10. Nurse Jones gives Pam positive feedback for attempting to make adaptive changes in her life.

CLINICAL EXPERIENCE

Have students keep a diary of relationship development with their patients in the clinical setting. They should identify each of the phases and the tasks that they have completed during each phase. The conditions essential to therapeutic relationship development (rapport, trust, respect, genuineness, and empathy) should all be considered. Discuss how their records compare and contrast with the textbook description of relationship development.

SIX SUBROLES OF NURSING

(Hildegard Peplau)

MOTHER-SURROGATE

TECHNICIAN

MANAGER

SOCIALIZING AGENT

HEALTH TEACHER

COUNSELOR OR PSYCHOTHERAPIST

CONDITIONS ESSENTIAL TO THERAPEUTIC RELATIONSHIP DEVELOPMENT

Rapport

Trust

Respect

Genuineness

Empathy

PHASES OF THERAPEUTIC NURSE-PATIENT RELATIONSHIP

THE PREINTERACTION PHASE

A. Obtain patient information
B. Examine own feelings, fears, and anxieties

THE ORIENTATION (INTRODUCTORY) PHASE

A. Establish trust and rapport
B. Establish contract for intervention
C. Assess, formulate nursing diagnoses, establish goals

THE WORKING PHASE

A. Maintain trust and rapport
B. Use problem-solving model
C. Overcome resistance
D. Continuously evaluate progress

THE TERMINATION PHASE

A. Goals have been achieved
B. A plan is established for continuing assistance
C. Feelings regarding termination are explored

CHAPTER 5: THERAPEUTIC COMMUNICATION

CHAPTER FOCUS

The focus of this chapter is to introduce the student to the concept of communication. Both verbal and nonverbal components of expression are discussed, and a description of therapeutic and nontherapeutic techniques is given.

LEARNING OBJECTIVES

After reading this chapter, the student will be able to:

1. Discuss the transactional model of communication.
2. Identify types of pre-existing conditions that influence the outcome of the communication process.
3. Define *territoriality, density and distance* as components of the environment.
4. Identify components of nonverbal expression.
5. Describe therapeutic and nontherapeutic verbal communication techniques.
6. Describe active listening.
7. Discuss therapeutic feedback.

KEY TERMS

territoriality   social distance
density   public distance
intimate distance   paralanguage
personal distance

CHAPTER OUTLINE/LECTURE NOTES

I. Introduction
   A. The nurse must be aware of the therapeutic or nontherapeutic value of the communication techniques used with the patient, for they are the "tools" of psychosocial intervention.
II. What is Communication?
   A. Interpersonal communication is a *transaction* between the sender and the receiver. Both persons participate simultaneously.
   B. In the transactional model, both participants are perceiving each other, listening to each other, and simultaneously engaged in the process of creating meaning in a relationship.
III. The Impact of Pre-existing Conditions
   A. Both sender and receiver bring certain pre-existing conditions to the exchange that influence both the intended message and the way in which it is interpreted.
      1. Values, attitudes, and beliefs. Examples: Attitudes of prejudice are expressed through negative stereotyping. A person who values youth may dress and behave in a manner that is characteristic of one who is much younger.
      2. Culture or religion. Cultural mores, norms, ideas, and customs provide the basis for our way of thinking. Examples: Men who hug each other on the street give a different message in the Italian culture than they would in the American culture. Some messages about religion are conveyed by wearing crosses around one's neck or hanging crucifixes on the wall.
      3. Social status. High status persons often convey their high-power position with gestures. Examples: less eye contact, more relaxed posture, louder voice pitch, more frequent use of hands on hips, power dressing, greater height, and more distance when communicating with individuals considered to be of lower social status.

4. Gender. Masculine and feminine gestures influence messages conveyed in communication with others. Examples: differences in posture and gender roles within various cultures.

5. Age or developmental level. Examples of developmental level on communication is especially evident during adolescence, with words such as cool, groovy, awesome, and others. Sign language is a unique system of gestures used by individuals who are deaf or hearing impaired.

6. Environment in which the transaction takes place. Territoriality, density, and distance are aspects of environment that communicate messages.
    a. Territoriality - the innate tendency to own space. All individuals lay claim to certain areas as their own, and feel safer in their own area.
    b. Density - the number of people within a given environmental space. Prolonged exposure to high density situations elicits certain behaviors, such as aggression, stress, criminal activity, and hostility.
    c. Distance - the means by which various cultures use space to communicate.
        (1) intimate distance - the closest distance that individuals will allow between themselves and others. In America, it is 0 to 18 inches.
        (2) personal distance - interactions that are personal in nature, such as close conversations with friends. In America, it is 18 to 40 inches.
        (3) social distance - conversations with strangers or acquaintances (e.g., at a cocktail party). In America, it is 4 to 12 feet.
        (4) public distance - speaking in public or yelling to someone some distance away. In America, the distance exceeds 12 feet.

IV. Nonverbal Communication
    A. Physical appearance and dress. Ways in which individuals dress or wear their hair conveys a message to all who observe the appearance. Example: unkept appearance may give an impression to some people that the individual is sloppy and irresponsible.
    B. Body movement and posture. The way in which an individual positions his or her body communicates messages regarding self-esteem, gender identity, status, and interpersonal warmth and coldness. Examples:
        1. Slumped posture, head and eyes pointed downward conveys a message of low self-esteem.
        2. Sitting with legs crossed at the thighs sometimes depicts feminine identity.
        3. Standing tall with head high and hands on hips indicates a superior status over the person being addressed.
        4. Warmth is conveyed by a smile, direct eye contact, and keeping the hands still.
    C. Touch. Can elicit both negative and positive reactions, depending upon cultural interpretation. Types of touch:
        1. Functional-professional: impersonal, business-like touch. Example: tailor fitting a suit.
        2. Social-polite: impersonal, but affirming. Example: a handshake.
        3. Friendship-warmth: indicates a strong liking for another person. Example: laying one's hand upon the shoulder of another.
        4. Love-intimacy: conveys an emotional attachment or attraction for another person. Example: to engage in a strong, mutual embrace.
        5. Sexual arousal: an expression of physical attraction. Example: touching another in the genital region.
    D. Facial expressions. Next to human speech, facial expression is the primary source of communication. The face can give multiple messages, such as happiness, sadness, anger, surprise, doubt, fear, disgust.
    E. Eye behavior. Eyes have been called the "windows of the soul." Social and cultural rules dictate where we can look, when we can look, for how long we can look, and at whom we can look. Eye contact conveys a personal interest in the other person. Staring or gazing can make another feel very uncomfortable.
    F. Vocal cues or paralanguage. Paralanguage is the gestural component of the spoken word. It consists of pitch, tone, and loudness of spoken messages, the rate of speaking, expressively placed pauses, and emphasis assigned to certain words. *How* a message is verbalized can be as important as *what* is verbalized.

V. Therapeutic Communication Techniques
    A. Using silence - allows the patient to take control of the discussion, if they so desire.
    B. Accepting - conveys positive regard.
    C. Giving recognition - acknowledging; indicating awareness.
    D. Offering self - making oneself available.
    E. Giving broad openings - allow patient to select the topic.
    F. Offering general leads - encourage patient to continue.
    G. Placing the event in time or sequence - clarifying the relationship of events in time.
    H. Making observations - verbalizing what is observed or perceived.
    I. Encouraging description of perceptions - asking the patient to verbalize what is being perceived.
    J. Encouraging comparison - asking patient to compare similarities and difference in ideas, experiences, or

interpersonal relationships.
- K. Restating - lets the patient know whether an expressed statement has been understood or not.
- L. Reflecting - questions or feelings are referred back to the patient so that they may be recognized and accepted.
- M. Focusing - taking notice of a single idea or even a single world.
- N. Exploring - delving further into a subject, idea, experience, or relationship.
- O. Seeking clarification and validation - striving to explain that which is vague and searching for mutual understanding.
- P. Presenting reality - clarifying misperceptions that the patient may be expressing.
- Q. Voicing doubt - expressing uncertainty as to the reality of the patient's perceptions.
- R. Verbalizing the implied - putting into words what the patient has only implied.
- S. Attempting to translate words into feelings - putting into words the feelings that patient has expressed only indirectly.
- T. Formulating a plan of action - strives to prevent anger or anxiety from escalating to an unmanageable level the next time the stressor occurs.

VI. Nontherapeutic Communication Techniques
- A. Giving reassurance - may discourage patient from further expression of feelings if he or she believes they will only be belittled.
- B. Rejecting - refusing to consider the patient's ideas or behavior.
- C. Giving approval or disapproval - implies that the nurse has the right to pass judgment on the "goodness" or "badness" of the patient's behavior.
- D. Agreeing/disagreeing - implies that the nurse has the right to pass judgment on whether the patient's ideas or opinions are "right or "wrong."
- E. Giving advice - implies that the nurse knows what is best for the patient, and that the patient is incapable of any self-direction.
- F. Probing - pushing for answers to issues the patient does not wish to discuss causes the patient to feel used and valued only for what is shared with the nurse.
- G. Defending - to defend what the patient has criticized implies that he or she has no right to express ideas, opinions, or feelings.
- H. Requesting an explanation - asking "Why?" implies that the patient must defend his or her behavior or feelings.
- I. Indicating the existence of an external source of power - encourages the patient to project blame for his or her thoughts or behaviors upon others.
- J. Belittling feelings expressed - causes the patient to feel insignificant or unimportant.
- K. Making stereotyped comments - cliches and trite expressions are meaningless in a nurse-patient relationship.
- L. Using denial - blocks discussion with the patient and avoids helping the patient identify and explore areas of difficulty.
- M. Interpreting - results in the therapist telling the patient the meaning of his experience.
- N. Introducing an unrelated topic - causes the nurse to take over the direction of the discussion.

VII. Active Listening
- A. To listen actively is to be attentive to what the patient is saying, both verbally, and nonverbally. Several nonverbal behaviors have been designed as facilitative skills for attentive listening. They can be identified by the acronym SOLER.
  1. S - Sit squarely facing the patient.
  2. O - Observe an open posture.
  3. L - Lean forward toward the patient.
  4. E - Establish eye contact.
  5. R - Relax.

VIII Feedback
- A. Feedback is useful when it is conveyed in the following manner:
  1. Feedback is descriptive rather than evaluative and focuses on the behavior rather than on the patient.
  2. Feedback should be specific rather than general.
  3. Feedback should be directed toward behavior that the patient has the capacity to modify.
  4. Feedback should impart information rather than offering advice.
  5. Feedback should be well-timed.

IX. Summary
X. Review Questions

LEARNING ACTIVITIES

INTERPERSONAL COMMUNICATION TECHNIQUES

After reading the communication on the left, indicate what technique the nurse has used, and whether the technique is therapeutic or nontherapeutic. Selections may be made from the list below. The first one has been completed as an example.

Giving recognition   Giving broad openings   Voicing doubt   Restating   Reflecting
Focusing   Verbalizing the implied   Exploring   Giving advice Rejecting
Giving reassurance   Indicating an external   Requesting an   Belittling   Defending
                        source of power   explanation   feelings

1. Pt: "The FBI wants to kill me."
   Ns: "I find that hard to believe."   ___Voicing doubt___   T   N

2. Ns Asst: "Mr. J. always calls me sweetie pie. I get so
   angry when he does that."
   Ns: "Perhaps you should consider how he is feeling."   _____   T   N

3. Pt: "My daddy always tucked me into bed at night."
   Ns: "I'd like to talk more about your relationship
   with your father."   _____   T   N

4. Ns to pt: "Good morning, Sue. I see you are
   wearing the hair bow you made in OT."   _____   T   N

5. Pt: "I didn't really mean it when I said I wanted
   to die."
   Ns: "What makes you say those kinds of things?"   _____   T   N

6. Pt: "Do you think I should get a divorce?"
   Ns: "What do you think would be best for you?"   _____   T   N

7. Pt: "Whenever I ask for a different therapy, my
   doctor just ignores me!"
   Ns: "I'm sure he knows what's best for you."   _____   T   N

8. Pt: "We always had such fun on holidays when I was
   growing up."
   Ns: "Tell me more about what it was like when you
   were a little girl."   _____   T   N

9. Pt: (Mute - refusing to talk)
   Ns: "It must have been a horrible experience for you
   being the only survivor of the automobile accident."   _____   T   N

10. Pt: "I don't think my life will ever be the same
    again."
    Ns: "Cheer up. Everything's going to be okay."   _____   T   N

11. Pt: "I feel like such a failure in the eyes of my
    family."
    Ns: "You feel as though you have let your
    family down."   _____   T   N

12. Pt: "Do you think I should leave home and get
an apartment of my own?"
Ns: "I think you would be much better off away
from your parents." _____ T N

13. Pt: "Good morning, nurse."
Ns: "Good morning, Patricia. What would you
like to talk about today?" _____ T N

14. Pt: "I'd like to talk about my relationship
with my boyfriend, Jack."
Ns: "Oh, let's don't talk about that. You talk
about that too much." _____ T N

15. Pt: "I want to call my husband."
Ns: "Why do you want to talk to him after the way
he treated you?" _____ T N

47

CLINICAL EXERCISE

Have students keep process recordings of their interpersonal communications with patients, identifying techniques employed, and whether their interactions were therapeutic or nontherapeutic.

CONDITIONS AFFECTING COMMUNICATION

Values, Attitudes and Beliefs

Culture or Religion

Social Status

Gender

Age or Developmental Level

Environment

NONVERBAL COMMUNICATION

Physical Appearance and Dress

Body Movement and Posture

Touch

Facial Expressions

Eye Behavior

Vocal Cues or Paralanguage

ACTIVE LISTENING

S - **Sit squarely facing the patient.**

O - **Observe an open posture.**

L - **Lean forward toward the patient.**

E - **Establish eye contact.**

R - **Relax.**

CHAPTER 6: THE NURSING PROCESS IN PSYCHIATRIC/MENTAL HEALTH NURSING

CHAPTER FOCUS

The focus of this chapter is to introduce the reader to each of the five steps of the nursing process. Documentation of the nursing process is also discussed.

LEARNING OBJECTIVES

After reading this chapter, the student will be able to:

1. Define nursing process.
2. Identify the five steps of the nursing process and describe nursing actions associated with each.
3. Describe the benefits of using nursing diagnosis.
4. Discuss the list of NANDA-accepted nursing diagnoses.
5. Apply the five steps of the nursing process in the care of a patient within the psychiatric setting.
6. Document patient care that validates use of the nursing process.

KEY TERMS

nursing process
nursing diagnosis
case management
critical pathways of care
diagnostic related group (DRG)

multidisciplinary
problem oriented recording
focus charting
PIE charting

CHAPTER OUTLINE/LECTURE NOTES

I. The Nursing Process
   A. A systematic framework for the delivery of nursing care.
   B. Uses a problem-solving approach.
   C. Is goal-directed: the delivery of quality patient care.
   D. Is dynamic, not static
      1. Assessment: information is gathered from which to establish a patient data base.
      2. Analysis: data from the assessment are analyzed; appropriate nursing diagnoses are selected from the data; and measurable outcome criteria are established.
      3. Plan: interventions for achieving the outcome criteria are selected.
      4. Implementation: interventions selected during the planning stage are executed.
      5. Evaluation: success of the interventions in meeting the outcome criteria is measured.
II. Why Nursing Diagnosis?
   A. Identification and classification of nursing phenomena began in 1973 with the First National Conference on Nursing Diagnosis
   B. Both general and specialty standards are written around the five steps of the nursing process, of which nursing diagnosis is an inherent part
   C. Defined in most state nurse practice acts as a legal responsibility of nursing
   D. Promotes research in nursing
III. Nursing Case Management
   A. Defined: a health care delivery process whose goals are to provide quality health care, decrease fragmentation, enhance the client's quality of life, and contain costs (ANA, 1988)

     B. Case Manager: coordinates the patient's care from admission to discharge, and in many cases, following discharge

     C. Critical Pathways: the tools for provision of care in a case management system. An abbreviated plan of care that provides outcome-based guidelines for goal achievement within a designated length of stay.

VI.   Applying Nursing Process in the Psychiatric Setting

     A. Role of the nurse in psychiatry

       1. To assist the patient to successfully adapt to stressors within the environment.

       2. Goals are directed toward change in thoughts, feelings, and behaviors that are age-appropriate and congruent with local and cultural norms.

       3. Nurses are a valuable member of the interdisciplinary team, providing a service that is unique and based on sound knowledge of psychopathology, scope of practice, and legal implications of the role.

V.   Documentation to the Nursing Process

     A. Documentation of the steps of the nursing is often considered as evidence in determining certain cases of negligence by nurses.

     B. Also required by some health care organization accrediting organizations.

     C. Examples of documentation that reflect use of the nursing process:

       1. Problem-Oriented Recording (POR)

         a. Has a list of problems as its basis

         b. Uses subjective, objective, assessment, plan, intervention, and evaluation (SOAPIE) format

       2. Focus Charting[R]

         a. Main perspective is to choose a "focus" for documentation. A focus may be:

           (1) a nursing diagnosis

           (2) a current patient concern or behavior

           (3) a significant change in the patient's status or behavior

           (4) a significant event in the patient's therapy

         b. The focus cannot be a medical diagnosis

         c. Uses a data, action, and response (DAR) format

       3. The "A PIE" method

         a. A problem-oriented system

         b. Utilizes flow sheets as accompanying documentation

         c. Uses an assessment, problem, intervention, and evaluation (A PIE) format

VI.   Summary

VII.   Review Questions

LEARNING ACTIVITIES

Read the following case study and follow the directions given below for application of the nursing process.

Case Study: Sam is presented through the emergency department to the psychiatric unit of a major medical center. He was taken to the hospital by local police who were called by department store security when Sam frightened shoppers by yelling loudly to "imaginary" people and threatening to harm anyone who came close to him.

On the psychiatric unit, Sam keeps to himself, and walks away when anyone approaches him. He talks and laughs to himself, and tilts his head to the side, as if listening. When the nurse attempts to talk to him, he shouts, "Get away from me. I know you are one of them!" He picks up a chair, as if to use it for protection.

Sam's appearance is unkempt. His clothes are dirty and wrinkled, his hair is oily and uncombed, and there is an obvious body odor about him. The physician admits Sam with a diagnosis of paranoid schizophrenia, and orders Thorazine and Cogentin on both a scheduled and prn basis.

1. Identify four segments of information from the assessment data that would be significant to nursing.

   a._____
   b._____
   c._____
   d._____

2. List the appropriate nursing diagnoses from analysis of the data described in question 1.

   a._____
   b._____
   c._____
   d._____

3. Provide outcome criteria for the four nursing diagnoses.

   a._____
   b._____
   c._____
   d._____

4. Select appropriate nursing interventions to achieve the outcome criteria.

CLINICAL EXERCISE

Have students present case studies in postconference of patients with whom they have been working in the clinical setting. Instruct them to use the five steps of the nursing process in their presentation. Rationale for selection of the nursing diagnoses and interventions should be a part of the presentation. Encourage discussion by the other students.

THE NURSING PROCESS

Assessment

Analysis

Planning

Implementation

Evaluation

DOCUMENTATION TO THE NURSING PROCESS

Nursing Process	Problem Oriented Recording	Focus Charting	A PIE Method
Assessment	Subjective/ Objective	Data	Assessment
Analysis	Assessment		Problem
Planning	Plan		
Implementation	Intervention	Action	Intervention
Evaluation	Evaluation	Response	Evaluation

CHAPTER 7: THERAPEUTIC GROUPS

CHAPTER FOCUS

The focus of this chapter is on the dynamics and functions of therapeutic groups. The role of the nurse in this type of intervention is also discussed.

LEARNING OBJECTIVES

After reading this chapter, the student will be able to:

1. Define a group.
2. Discuss eight functions of a group.
3. Identify various types of groups.
4. Describe physical conditions that influence groups.
5. Discuss "curative factors" that occur in groups.
6. Describe the phase of group development.
7. Identify various leadership styles in groups.
8. Identify various roles that members assume within a group.
9. Discuss psychodrama and family therapy as specialized forms of group therapy.
10. Describe the role of the nurse in group therapy.

KEY TERMS

universality	psychodrama
altruism	group therapy
catharsis	therapeutic groups
autocratic	family therapy
laissez-faire	genogram

CHAPTER OUTLINE/LECTURE NOTES

I. The Group, Defined
    A. A collection of individuals whose association is founded upon shared commonalities of interest, values, norms, or purpose.
II. Functions of a Group
    A. Socialization - the teaching of social norms.
    B. Support - fellow members are available in time of need.
    C. Task Completion - assistance is provided when completion is enhanced by group involvement.
    D. Camaraderie - individuals receive joy and pleasure from interactions with significant others.
    E. Informational - learning takes place when group members share their knowledge with the others in the group.
    F. Normative - different groups enforce the established norms in various ways.
    G. Empowerment - change can be effected by groups at times when individuals alone are ineffective.
    H. Governance - large organizations often have leadership that is provided by groups rather than a single individual.
III. Types of Groups
    A. Task groups - a group formed to accomplish a specific outcome.
    B. Teaching groups - focus is to convey knowledge and information to a number of individuals.
    C. Supportive/therapeutic groups - the concern of these groups is to prevent possible future upsets by educating. the participants in effective ways of dealing with emotional stress arising from situational or developmental

crises.
  IV. Therapeutic Groups vs. Group Therapy
    A. Group therapy has a sound theoretical base and their leaders generally have advanced degrees in psychology, social work, nursing, or medicine.
    B. Therapeutic groups are based to a lesser degree in theory. Focus is on group relations, interactions between group members, and the consideration of a selected issue.
    C. Leaders of both types of groups must be knowledgeable about group *process* (the way in which group members interact with each other), as well as group *content* (the topic or issue being discussed in the group).
  V. Physical Conditions that Influence Group Dynamics
    A. Seating - it is best when there is no barrier between the members. For example, a circle of chairs is better than chairs set around a table.
    B. Size - size of the group makes a difference in the interaction among members. Seven or eight members provides a favorable climate for optimal group interaction and relationship development.
    C. Membership - two types of groups exist: open ended groups (those in which members leave and others join at any time during the existence of the group) and closed ended groups (those in which all members join at the time the group is organized and terminate at the end of the designated length of time).
  VI. Curative Factors
    A. The instillation of hope. By observing the progress of others in the group with similar problems, a group member garners hope that his or her problems can also be resolved.
    B. Universality. Individuals come to realize that they are not alone in the problems, thoughts, and feelings they are experiencing.
    C. The imparting of information. Group members share their knowledge with each other. Leaders of teaching groups also provide information to group members.
    D. Altruism. Individuals provide assistance and support to each other, thereby creating a positive self-image and promoting self-growth.
    E. The corrective recapitulation of the primary family group. Group members are able to re-experience early family conflicts that remain unresolved.
    F. The development of socializing techniques. Through interaction with, and feedback from, other members within the group, individuals are able to correct maladaptive social behaviors and learn and develop new social skills.
    G. Imitative behavior. Group members who have mastered a particular psychosocial skill or developmental task serve as valuable role models for others.
    H. Interpersonal learning. The group offers many and varied opportunities for interacting with other people.
    I. Group cohesiveness. Members develop a sense of belonging that separates the individual ("I am") from the group ("we are").
    J. Catharsis. Within the group, members are able to express both positive and negative feelings.
    K. Existential factors. The group is able to assist individual members to take direction of their own lives and to accept responsibility for the quality of their existence.
  VII. Phases of Group Development
    A. Initial or orientation phase
      1. Leader and members work together to establish rules and goals for the group.
      2. The leader promotes trust and ensures that the rules do not interfere with the fulfillment of the goals.
      3. Members are superficial and overly polite. Trust has not yet been established.
    B. Middle or working phase
      1. Productive work toward completion of the task is undertaken.
      2. Leader role diminishes and becomes more one of facilitator.
      3. Trust has been established between the members and cohesiveness exists. Conflict is managed by the group members themselves.
    C. Final or termination phase
      1. A sense of loss, precipitating the grief process, may be experienced by group members.
      2. The leader encourages the group members to discuss these feelings of loss, and to reminisce about the accomplishments of the group.
      3. Feelings of abandonment may be experienced by some members. Grief for previous losses may be triggered.
  VIII Leadership Styles
    A. Autocratic - the focus is on the leader, on whom the members are dependent for problem-solving, decision making, and permission to perform. Production is high, but morale is low.

LEARNING ACTIVITIES

FAMILY GENOGRAM

Have students construct their own genogram depicting three generations of their family. Encourage use of appropriate symbols to identify intensity and appropriateness of certain relationships. Have them follow the graphic depiction with a narrative explanation of family dynamics.

GROUP ATTENDANCE

Allow students to use clinical time to attend various types of groups. Following attendance, students should report back to the clinical group in terms of:

1. type of group attended (task, teaching, or supportive/therapeutic)
2. type of leadership identified for the group (give rationale for determination)
3. member roles identified (task roles, maintenance roles, personal roles)
4. description of group dynamics

Suggestions for possible group attendance include:

1. Task groups:
   a. various hospital committees
   b. interdisciplinary treatment team meetings
   c. nursing faculty curriculum committee meeting
   d. discharge planning meetings
2. Teaching groups:
   a. prepared childbirth classes
   b. diabetes education classes
   c. daily living skills groups
   d. medication classes
   e. transition to discharge groups
3. Supportive/therapeutic groups
   a. Alcoholics Anonymous
   b. Al-Anon
   c. Parents Without Partners
   d. Weight Watchers
   e. Overeaters Anonymous
   f. Widows Support Group
   g. Victims of Sexual Assault Support Group

TYPES OF GROUPS

Task Groups

Teaching Groups

Supportive/Therapeutic Groups

PHASES OF GROUP DEVELOPMENT

I. **INITIAL OR ORIENTATION PHASE**

   a. Establish rules and goals for the group
   b. Leader promotes environment of trust
   c. Members superficial and overly polite

II. **MIDDLE OR WORKING PHASE**

   a. Work toward task completion undertaken
   b. Leader becomes facilitator
   c. Members manage own conflict

III. **FINAL OR TERMINATION PHASE**

   a. Sense of loss may precipitate grief response
   b. Leader encourages review of group's work and expression of feelings
   c. Members generalize skills learned in group to other areas of their life

LEADERSHIP STYLES

AUTOCRATIC

    a. Focus: on the leader
    b. Limited member participation
    c. High productivity; low morale

DEMOCRATIC

    a. Focus: on the members
    b. Unlimited member participation
    c. High productivity; high morale

LAISSEZ-FAIRE

    a. Focus: undetermined
    b. Inconsistent member participation
    c. Low productivity; low morale

CHAPTER 8: MILIEU THERAPY - THE THERAPEUTIC COMMUNITY

CHAPTER FOCUS

The focus of this chapter is to introduce the student to the concept of milieu therapy. The role of the nurse in this therapeutic setting is emphasized.

LEARNING OBJECTIVES

After reading this chapter, the student will be able to:

1. Define *milieu therapy.*
2. Explain the goal of therapeutic community/milieu therapy.
3. Identify seven basic assumptions of a therapeutic community.
4. Discuss conditions that characterize a therapeutic community.
5. Identify the various therapies that may be included within the program of therapeutic community, and the health care workers that make up the interdisciplinary treatment team.
6. Describe the role of the nurse on the interdisciplinary treatment team.

KEY TERMS

milieu   therapeutic community
milieu therapy

CHAPTER OUTLINE/LECTURE NOTES

I.   Defined
     A. Milieu therapy or therapeutic community is defined as a scientific structuring of the environment in order to effect behavioral changes and to improve the psychological health and functioning of the individual.
     B. Within the therapeutic community setting, the patient is expected to learn adaptive coping, interaction and relationship skills that can be generalized to other aspects of his or her life.
II. Basic Assumptions
     A. The health in each individual is to be realized and encouraged to grow.
     B. Every interaction is an opportunity for therapeutic intervention.
     C. The patient owns his own environment.
     D. Each patient owns his behavior.
     E. Peer pressure is a useful and a powerful tool.
     F. Inappropriate behaviors are dealt with as they occur.
     G. Restrictions and punishment are to be avoided.
III. Conditions that Promote a Therapeutic Community
     A. Basic physiological needs are fulfilled.
     B. The physical facilities are conducive to achievement of the goals of therapy.
     C. A democratic form of self-government exists.
     D. Unit responsibilities are assigned according to patient capabilities.
     E. A structured program of social and work-related activities is scheduled as part of the treatment program.
     F. Community and family are included in the program of therapy in an effort to facilitate discharge from the hospital.
IV. The Program of Therapeutic Community
     A. Directed by an interdisciplinary team.
     B. A treatment plan is formulated by the team.

C. All disciplines sign the treatment plan and meet weekly to update the plan as needed.

D. Disciplines may include psychiatry, psychology, nursing, social work, occupational therapy, recreational therapy, art therapy, music therapy, dietetics, and chaplain service.

V.   Role of the Nurse

A. The ANA standards state, "The nurse provides, structures, and maintains a therapeutic environment in collaboration with the client and other health care providers."

B. Through use of the nursing process, nursing manages the therapeutic environment on a 24-hour basis.

C. Nurses have the responsibility for ensuring that patients' physiological and psychological needs are met.

D. Nurses also are responsible for:

1. medication administration
2. development of a one-to-one relationship
3. setting limits on unacceptable behavior
4. patient education

VI. Summary

VII. Review Questions

LEARNING ACTIVITIES

Identify the appropriate member of the interdisciplinary for the activity listed. Choices may be made from the following list.

psychiatrist	staff nurse	art therapist
clinical psychologist	occupational therapist	dietitian
social worker	recreational therapist	chaplain
clinical nurse specialist	music therapist	

1. Accompanies patients to see a movie.
   _____

2. Helps patients identify unconscious feelings through their drawings.
   _____

3. Conducts psychological testing to assist the psychiatrist to determine a correct diagnosis.
   _____

4. Serves the spiritual needs of psychiatric patients.
   _____

5. Monitors nutritional needs for patient with special requirements.
   _____

6. Teaches relaxation techniques through the use of music.
   _____

7. Conducts assertiveness training.
   _____

8. Prescribes electroconvulsive therapy for a depressed patient.
   _____

9. Administers medication.
   _____

10. Locates appropriate placement for the patient following hospital discharge.
   _____

11. Assists patients to increase self-esteem by providing small craft items for completion and display.
   _____

There are seven basic assumptions upon which a therapeutic community is based. Identify the assumption (from the column on the right) that is the foundation for each of the situations listed on the left.

_____ 1. John came into the TV room and changed the channel in the middle of a program that several others were watching. The group reprimanded him loudly, and returned the TV to the channel they had been watching. They told him they would not tolerate that kind of behavior.

_____ 2. Even though she seemed unable to change, Nancy had a great deal of insight into her own behavior. She knew it was maladaptive and she knew it had psychological implications. The nurse focused on Nancy's insight and knowledge to help her find more adaptive ways of coping.

_____ 3. George always started an argument in group therapy. Each time, the group calmed him down with their discussion. However, when he became violent, he was placed in isolation for the safety of himself and others.

_____ 4. Fred becomes angry whenever anyone in the group disagrees with him. Members of the group examine Fred's defensiveness, and help him to see how he is coming across to others. They help him to practice more appropriate ways of responding.

_____ 5. Lloyd had always been unable to interact on a personal level with other people. In the milieu environment, he learned new communication skills and had the opportunity to practice relationship development that helped him when he left the hospital.

_____ 6. Kevin told the nurse of being arrested for driving the getaway car in an armed robbery. He stated, "I don't know why they grabbed me. Jack did the stealing! He made me drive the car." The nurse responded, "Kevin, no one made you drive the car. You made that choice yourself. Now you must own up to that decision."

_____ 7. Carol was elected unit president at the community meeting. She assigns chores for the week, and calls for a vote concerning late privileges for patients on Saturday night.

a. The health in each individual is to be realized and encouraged to grow.

b. Every interaction is an opportunity for therapeutic intervention.

c. The patient owns his own environment.

d. Each patient owns his behavior.

e. Peer pressure is a useful and powerful tool.

f. Inappropriate behavior is dealt with as it occurs.

g. Restrictions and punishment are to be avoided.

BASIC ASSUMPTIONS ON WHICH THERAPEUTIC MILIEU IS BASED

1. The Health In Each Individual Is To Be Realized And Encouraged to Grow.

2. Every Interaction Is An Opportunity For Therapeutic Intervention.

3. The Patient Owns His Own Environment.

4. Each Patient Owns His Behavior.

5. Peer Pressure Is A Useful And Powerful Tool.

6. Inappropriate Behaviors Are Dealt With As They Occur.

7. Restrictions And Punishment Are To Be Avoided.

THE INTERDISCIPLINARY TREATMENT TEAM

Psychiatrist

Clinical Psychologist

Psychiatric Social Worker

Clinical Nurse Specialist

Staff Nurse

Mental Health Technician

Occupational Therapist

Recreational Therapist

Music Therapist

Art Therapist

Psychodramatist

Dietitian

Chaplain

CHAPTER 9: CRISIS INTERVENTION

CHAPTER FOCUS

The focus of this chapter is to introduce the student to the concept of crisis, and the therapy of crisis intervention. The role of the nurse in crisis intervention is emphasized.

LEARNING OBJECTIVES

After reading this chapter, the student will be able to:

1. Define *crisis*.
2. Describe four phases in the development of a crisis.
3. Identify types of crises that occur in people's lives.
4. Discuss the goal of crisis intervention.
5. Describe the steps in crisis intervention.
6. Identify the role of the nurse in crisis intervention.

KEY TERMS

crisis
crisis intervention

CHAPTER OUTLINE/LECTURE NOTES

I. Definition
   A. Crisis has been defined as a psychological disequilibrium in a person who confronts a hazardous circumstance that for him constitutes an important problem which he can, for the time being, neither escape nor solve with his customary problem-solving resources.
   B. Assumptions upon which the concept of crisis is based.
      1. Crisis occurs in all individuals at one time or another and is not necessarily equated with psychopathology.
      2. Crises are precipitated by specific identifiable events.
      3. Crises are personal by nature.
      4. Crises are acute, not chronic, and will be resolved in one way or another within a brief period of time.
      5. A crisis situation contains the potential for psychological growth or deterioration.
II. Phases in the Development of a Crisis
   A. The individual is exposed to a precipitating stressor.
   B. When previous problem-solving techniques do not relieve the stressor, anxiety increases further.
   C. All possible resources, both internal and external, are called upon to resolve the problem and relieve the discomfort.
   D. If resolution does not occur in previous phases, the tension mounts beyond a further threshold or its burden increases over time to a breaking point. Major disorganization of the individual, with drastic results, often occurs.
III. Types of Crises
   A. Dispositional crisis - an acute response to an external situational stressor.
   B. Crisis of anticipated life transitions - normal life cycle transitions that may be anticipated, but over which the individual may feel a lack of control.
   C. Crisis resulting from traumatic stress - a crisis that is precipitated by an unexpected, external stressor over which the individual has little or no control, and from which he or she feels emotionally overwhelmed and defeated.

71

D. Maturational/developmental crisis - crisis that occurs in response to situations that trigger emotions related to unresolved conflicts in one's life.

E. Crisis reflecting psychopathology - emotional crisis in which pre-existing psychopathology has been instrumental in precipitating the crisis or in which psychopathology significantly impairs or complicates adaptive resolution.

F. Psychiatric emergencies - crisis situations in which general functioning has been severely impaired and the individual rendered incompetent or unable to assume personal responsibility.

IV. Crisis Intervention

A. The minimum therapeutic goal of crisis intervention is psychological resolution of the individual's immediate crisis and restoration to at least the level of functioning that existed before the crisis period.

B. A maximum goal is improvement in functioning above the precrisis level.

C. Usually lasts from 4 to 6 weeks.

V. Phases of Crisis Intervention: The Role of the Nurse

A. Nurses may be called upon to function as crisis helpers in virtually any setting committed to the practice of nursing.

1. Assessment. Information is gathered regarding the precipitating stressor and the resulting crisis that prompted the individual to seek professional help.

2. Analysis. From the assessment data, the nurse selects appropriate nursing diagnoses that reflect the immediacy of the crisis situation. Desired outcome criteria are established.

3. Planning. Appropriate nursing actions are selected, taking into consideration the type of crisis, as well as the individual's strengths, and available resources for support.

4. Intervention. The actions identified in the planning phase are implemented. A reality-oriented approach is used. A rapid working relationship is established by showing unconditional acceptance, by active listening, and by attending to immediate needs. A problem-solving model becomes the basis for change.

5. Evaluation. A reassessment is conducted to determine if the stated objectives were achieved. A plan of action is developed for the individual to deal with the stressor, should it recur.

VI. Summary

VII. Review Questions

LEARNING ACTIVITIES

Match the situation on the left with the type of crisis listed on the right.

_____ 1. 24-year-old Harriet was informed that her husband was killed in an industrial accident at the plant where he works. An hour later, she was found walking down a busy highway saying, "I'm looking for my lucky rabbit's foot. Everything will be okay if I can just find my luck rabbit's foot."

_____ 2. Ted was transferred on his job to a distant city. His wife, Jane, had never lived away from her family before. She became despondent, living only for daily phone calls to her relatives back in their home town.

_____ 3. Carrie knew when she married Matt that he had a drinking problem, but she believed he would change. Last night, after becoming intoxicated, Matt beat Carrie into unconsciousness. When she regained consciousness, he was gone. She took a taxi to the emergency department of the local hospital.

_____ 4. Linda had a history of obsessive-compulsive disorder. She was phobic about germs, and washed her hands many times every day. Last night, after a party, she had sex with a fellow college student she barely knew. Today, she is extremely anxious, and keeps repeating that she knows she has AIDS. Her roommate cannot get her to come out of the shower.

_____ 5. At age 13, Sue was raped by her uncle. The abuse continued for several years. He threatened to kill her mother if she told. Sue is 23 years old now, and recently became engaged. She has never had an intimate relationship, and experiences panic attacks at the thought of her wedding night.

_____ 6. Frank was very proud of his home. He had saved for many years to build it, and had virtually built it from the ground up by himself. Last night, while he and his wife were visiting a nearby town, a tornado ripped through his neighborhood and totally destroyed his home. Frank is devastated, and for over a week has sat and stared into space, barely eating and rarely speaking.

a. dispositional crisis

b. crisis of anticipated life transition

c. crisis resulting from traumatic stress

d. maturational/developmental crisis

e. crisis reflecting psychopathology

f. psychiatric emergencies

73

You are a nurse in the mental health clinic in the town to which Ted and Jane (situation #2 in the previous activity) have moved. Ted brings Jane to your clinic and explains that she has become nonfunctional since their move. Use the steps of the problem-solving process with the objective of assisting Jane to overcome her despondency.

1. Confront the problem.

2. Identify realistic changes.

3. Explore coping strategies for aspects about her situation that cannot be changed.

4. Identify various alternatives for coping with the situation.

5. Weigh benefits and consequences of each alternative.

6. Select most appropriate alternative.

PHASES IN DEVELOPMENT OF A CRISIS

PHASE 1: The individual is exposed to a precipitating stressor.

PHASE 2: When previous problem-solving techniques do not relieve the stressor, anxiety increases further.

PHASE 3: All possible resources, both internal and external, are called upon to resolve the problem and relieve the discomfort.

PHASE 4: Tension mounts and, over time, increases to the breaking point. The individual experiences major disorganization.

TYPES OF CRISES

Dispositional Crises

Crises of Anticipated Life Transitions

Crises Resulting From Traumatic Stress

Maturational/Developmental Crises

Crises Reflecting Psychopathology

Psychiatric Emergencies

CHAPTER 10: RELAXATION THERAPY

CHAPTER FOCUS

The focus of this chapter is to introduce the student to the benefits of relaxation therapy. Various methods of achieving relaxation are presented, and emphasis is on the role of the nurse in relaxation therapy.

LEARNING OBJECTIVES

After reading this chapter, the student will be able to:

1.   Identify conditions for which relaxation is appropriate therapy.
2.   Describe physiological and behavioral manifestations of relaxation.
3.   Discuss various methods of achieving relaxation.
4.   Describe the role of the nurse in relaxation therapy.

KEY TERMS

stress management   mental imagery
progressive relaxation   biofeedback
meditation

CHAPTER OUTLINE/LECTURE NOTES

I.   The Stress Epidemic
      A. Stress is rapidly permeating our society.
      B. Individuals experience the "fight or flight" response on a regular basis.
      C. The "fight or flight" emergency response is inappropriate to today's psychosocial stresses that persist over long periods of time.
      D. Stress is known to be a major contributor, either directly or indirectly, to coronary heart disease, cancer, lung ailments, accidental injuries, cirrhosis of the liver, and suicide--six of the leading causes of death in the United States.
      E. An individual's predisposing factors (genetic influences, past experiences, and existing conditions) influence the degree of severity to which an individual perceives and responds to stress.
II.   Physiological, Cognitive, and Behavioral Manifestations of Relaxation
      A. Physiological manifestations of stress include increases in heart rate, respiration, blood pressure, blood sugar, and metabolism.
      B. Behavioral manifestations of stress include restlessness, irritability, insomnia, and anorexia.
      C. Cognitive manifestations of stress include confusion, and difficulty with concentration, problem-solving, and learning.
      D. Relaxation can counteract these symptoms.
III. Methods of Achieving Relaxation
      A. Deep breathing exercises
          1. Relaxation is accomplished by allowing the lungs to breathe in as much oxygen as possible. Air is breathed in slowly through the nose, held for a few seconds, and then exhaled slowly through the mouth.
          2. Breathing exercises have been found to be effective in reducing anxiety, depression, irritability, muscular tension, and fatigue.
          3. An advantage of this type of exercise is that it may be accomplished anywhere at any time.
      B. Progressive relaxation
          1. Each muscle group is tensed for 5 to 7 seconds, and then relaxed for 20 to 30 seconds, during which time

the individual concentrates on the difference in sensations between the two conditions.
2. Excellent results have been observed with this method in the treatment of muscular tension, anxiety, insomnia, depression, fatigue, irritable bowel, muscle spasms, neck and back pain, high blood pressure, mild phobias, and stuttering.
C. Modified (or passive) progressive relaxation
1. Relaxation is achieved with this method by passively concentrating on the feeling of relaxation within the muscle.
D. Meditation
1. Meditation has been practiced for over 2000 years.
2. The goal of meditation is to gain "mastery over attention."
3. Relaxation is achieved through achievement of a special state of consciousness brought on by extreme concentration solely on one thought or object.
4. It has been used successfully in the treatment of cardiovascular disease, obsessive thinking, anxiety, depression, and hostility.
E. Mental imagery
1. This method of relaxation employs the imagination in an effort to reduce the body's response to stress.
2. The individual follows his or her imagination in selecting an environment considered to be relaxing.
3. The individual then concentrates on this relaxing image in an effort to achieve relaxation.
4. Soft, background music enhances the effect.
F. Biofeedback
1. Biofeedback is the use of instrumentation to become aware of processes in the body that usually go unnoticed, and to help bring them under to voluntary control. Some of these processes include blood pressure, muscle tension, skin surface temperature, and heart rate.
2. Biofeedback has been used successfully in the treatment of spastic colon, hypertension, tension and migraine headaches, muscle spasms/pain, anxiety, phobias, stuttering, and teeth grinding.
G. Physical exercise
1. Physical exertion provides a natural outlet for the tension produced by the body in its state of arousal for "fight or flight."
2. Following exercise, physiological equilibrium is restored resulting in a feeing of relaxation and revitalization.
3. Aerobic exercises have been shown to be successful in strengthening the cardiovascular system.
4. Low intensity physical exercise can help prevent obesity, relieve muscular tension, prevent muscle spasms, and increase flexibility.
5. Physical exercise can also be effective in reducing general anxiety and depression.
IV. Role of the Nurse in Relaxation Therapy
A. Nurses can help individuals recognize the source of stress in their lives and identify methods of adaptive coping.
B. Nurses can serve as educators to increase patients' knowledge regarding methods for achieving relaxation.
C. Relaxation therapy provides alternatives to old, maladaptive methods of coping with stress.
D. Nurses can help individuals analyze the usefulness of various relaxation techniques in the management of stress in their daily lives.
V. Summary
VI. Review Questions

LEARNING ACTIVITIES

Take the following self-test. Discuss the results in class or small student groups.

How Vulnerable Are You To Stress?

Score each item from 1 (almost always) to 5 (never), according to how much of the time each statement applies to you.

____ 1. I eat at least one hot, balanced meal day.
____ 2. I get 7 to 8 hours of sleep at least 4 nights a week.
____ 3. I give and receive affection regularly.
____ 4. I have at least one relative within 50 miles on whom I can rely.
____ 5. I exercise to the point of perspiration at least twice a week.
____ 6. I smoke less than half a pack of cigarettes a day.
____ 7. I take fewer than five alcoholic drinks a week.
____ 8. I am the appropriate weight for my height.
____ 9. I have an income adequate to meet basic expenses.
____ 10. I get strength from my religious beliefs.
____ 11. I regularly attend club or social activities.
____ 12. I have a network of friends and acquaintances.
____ 13. I have one or more friends to confide in about personal matters.
____ 14. I am in good health (including eyesight, hearing, teeth.)
____ 15. I am able to speak openly about my feelings when angry or worried.
____ 16. I have regular conversations with the people I live with about domestic problems, e.g., chores,money, and daily living issues.
____ 17. I do something for fun at least once a week.
____ 18. I am able to organize my time effectively.
____ 19. I drink fewer than 3 cups of coffee (or tea or colas) a day.
____ 20. I take quiet time for myself during the day.

____ TOTAL

To get your score, add up the figures and subtract 20. Any number over 30 indicates a vulnerability to stress. You are seriously vulnerable if your score is between 50 and 75, and extremely vulnerable if it is over 75.

Keep a record for one week of situations that produce stress in your life. Rate the severity of each situation on a scale of 1 to 5 (with 5 being the most severe). Describe how you responded to the stress and whether your response was adaptive or maladaptive. If it was maladaptive, how could you have responded more adaptively?

Date	Situation	Rating (1-5)	How I Responded	Adaptive/ Maladaptive	How to respond adaptively

CLINICAL EXERCISE

Teach a relaxation exercise to a patient. Why was this particular exercise chosen for this individual? How and when will the patient use this exercise in his or her daily life style?

METHODS OF ACHIEVING RELAXATION

Deep Breathing Exercises

Progressive Relaxation

Modified (Passive) Progressive Relaxation

Meditation

Mental Imagery

Biofeedback

Physical Exercise

CHAPTER 11: ASSERTIVENESS TRAINING

CHAPTER FOCUS

The focus of this chapter is to introduce the student to the concepts of assertiveness training. Various techniques to promote assertive behavior are discussed, and the role of the nurse in assertiveness training is emphasized.

LEARNING OBJECTIVES

After reading this chapter, the student will be able to:

1. Define assertive behavior.
2. Discuss basic human rights.
3. Differentiate between nonassertive, assertive, aggressive and passive-aggressive behaviors.
4. Describe techniques that promote assertive behavior.
5. Demonstrate thought stopping techniques.
6. Discuss the role of the nurse in assertiveness training.

KEY TERMS

assertiveness

nonassertiveness

aggressiveness

passive-aggressiveness

thought-stopping

CHAPTER OUTLINE/LECTURE NOTES

I. Assertive Communication
    A. Assertiveness is behavior that enables individuals to act in their own best interests, to stand up for themselves without undue anxiety, to express their honest feelings comfortably, or to exercise their own rights without denying the rights of others.
    B. Honesty is basic to assertive behavior and is expressed in a manner that promotes self-respect and respect for others.
II. Basic Human Rights
    A. The right to be treated with respect.
    B. The right to express feelings, opinions, and beliefs.
    C. The right to say "no" without feeling guilty.
    D. The right to make mistakes and accept the responsibility for them.
    E. The right to be listened to, and taken seriously.
    F. The right to change one's mind.
    G. The right to ask for what you want.
    H. The right to put yourself first, sometimes.
    I. The right to set one's own priorities.
    J. The right to refuse justification for one's feelings or behavior.
    K. If one is to accept these rights, he or she must also accept the responsibilities that accompany them.
III. Response Patterns
    A. Individuals to develop, in certain ways, patterns of responding to others. These ways include:
        1. By watching other people (role modeling).
        2. By being positively reinforced or punished for a certain response.
        3. By inventing a response.
        4. By not thinking of a better way to respond

     5.   By not developing the proper skills for a better response.

     6.   By consciously choosing a response style

  B. Four common response patterns

     1.   Nonassertive behavior. Sometimes called passive, these individuals seek to please others at the expense of denying their own basic human rights.

     2.   Assertive behavior. These individuals stand up for their own rights while protecting the rights of others. Feelings are expressed openly and honestly. Self-respect and respect for others are maintained.

     3.   Aggressive behavior. These individuals defend their own basic rights by violating the basic rights of others. Aggressive behavior hinders interpersonal relationships.

     4.   Passive-aggressive behavior. These individuals defend their own rights by expressing resistance to social and occupational demands. Sometimes called *indirect aggression,* this behavior takes the form of passive, non-confrontive action. These individuals use actions instead of words to convey their message, and the actions express covert aggression.

IV.   Behavioral Components of Assertive Behavior

  A. Intermittent eye contact.

  B. Body posture: sitting and leaning slightly toward the other person in a conversation.

  C. Distance/physical contact: appropriate physical distance is culturally determined. Invasion of personal space may be interpreted by some individuals as aggressive.

  D. Gestures - may also be culturally related. Gestures can add meaning to the spoken word.

  E. Facial expression - various facial expressions convey different messages.

  F. Voice - the voice conveys a message by its loudness, softness, degree and placement of emphasis, and evidence of emotional tone.

  G. Fluency - being able to discuss a subject with ease and with obvious knowledge conveys assertiveness and self-confidence.

  H. Timing - assertive responses are most effective when they are spontaneous and immediate.

  I. Listening - assertive listening means giving the other individual full attention.

  J. Thoughts - one's attitudes about the appropriateness of assertive behavior influences one's responses.

  K. Content - many times it is not what is being said that is as important as how it is said.

V.   Techniques that Promote Assertive Behavior

  A. Standing up for one's basic human rights.

  B. Assuming responsibility for own statements.

  C. Responding as a "Broken Record." Persistently repeating in a calm voice what is wanted.

  D. Agreeing assertively. Assertively accepting negative aspects about oneself. Admitting when an error has been made.

  E. Inquiring assertively. Seeking additional information about critical statements.

  F. Shifting from content to process. Changing the focus of the communication from discussing the topic at hand to analyzing what is actually going on in the interaction.

  G. Clouding/fogging. Concurring with the critic's argument without becoming defensive and without agreeing to change.

  H. Defusing. Putting off further discussion with an angry individual until he or she is calmer.

  I. Delaying assertively. Putting off further discussion with another individual until one is calmer.

  J. Responding assertively with irony.

VI.   Thought-Stopping Techniques

  A. A technique that was developed to eliminate intrusive, unwanted thoughts.

  B. The individual practices interrupting negative thought processes with the word "stop," and shifting his or her thoughts to one that is considered pleasant and desirable.

VII. Role of the Nurse

  A. Nurses must understand and utilize assertive skills in order to effect change that will improve the status of nursing, and the system of health care provision in our country.

  B. Nurses who understand and use assertiveness skills themselves can, in turn, assist patients who wish to effect behavioral change to increase self-esteem and improve interpersonal relationships.

  C. Nurses can teach patients assertive skills on a one-to-one basis or in a group situation.

  D. Information should include examples of various behavioral responses (assertive, nonassertive, aggressive, and passive-aggressive), as well as techniques that can be used to promote assertive behavior.

  E. Patients should be given the opportunity to practice their newly learned skills through role play, in order to facilitate the behavior when the actual situation arises.

VIII. Summary

IX.   Review Questions

LEARNING ACTIVITIES

Match the responses on the left to the assertive technique being used.

_____ 1. Wife: "You let that guy walk all over you. What a wimp!"
Husband: "Yes, I admit I didn't handle that situation very well."

_____ 2. Husband: "Would you please re-sew this seam. It's coming loose again."
Wife: "I can never do anything to please you!"
Husband: "Seems we need to discuss the real issue here."

_____ 3. Man: "If I were your husband, I'd keep my eye on you all the time.
Woman: "It's so nice to know you care."

_____ 4. Man Board Member: "How dare you suggest we hire homosexuals! What kind of company do you think this is?"
Woman Board Member: "I would like to discuss this further with you when you have had a chance to cool off."

_____ 5. Woman #1: "How can you be in favor of abortion? Can't you see it's murder?"
Woman #2: "I have a right to my opinion just as you have."

_____ 6. Door-to-door salesman: "I'd like to demonstrate this steam cleaner by cleaning one of your rugs for you."
Housewife: "I'm not interested in seeing a demonstration of a steam cleaner."
Door-to-door salesman: "But surely you have a rug you'd like to have cleaned!"
Housewife: "I'm not interested in seeing a demonstration of a steam cleaner."

_____ 7. Husband: "Boy, I can't believe you screwed up that audition so badly."
Wife: "Just what do you think I did that was so wrong?"

_____ 8. Male staff nurse: "I think the changes I have proposed for the unit will improve staff relations, not to mention patient care. I'm surprised they haven't been thought of before."
Female head nurse: "Thank you for your suggestions. I will study them and talk to you about them later."

a. Standing up for one's basic human rights.

b. Assuming responsibility for own statements.

c. Responding as a "broken record."

d. Agreeing assertively.

e. Inquiring assertively

f. Shifting from content to process.

g. Clouding/fogging.

h. Defusing

i. Delaying assertively.

j. Responding assertively with irony.

_____ 9. Husband: If you'd just slow down, you wouldn't make so many mistakes!"
Wife: "You are probably right. It probably would help if I slowed down some."

_____ 10. Head Nurse: "I need someone to stay on and work an extra shift."
Staff Nurse: "I don't want to work an extra shift tonight."

ROLE PLAY

Have students rate their behavior on the assertiveness evaluation tool presented in the text (Figure 11.1). Instruct them to identify areas in which they could be more assertive. Have them practice increasing their assertive skills by role playing situations in small groups that represent areas in which they rated themselves as nonassertive on the tool. This may also be accomplished in larger groups, by asking the observers to critique the responses given in role play.

BASIC ASSERTIVE HUMAN RIGHTS

1. The right to be treated with respect.

2. The right to express feelings, opinions, and beliefs.

3. The right to say "no" without feeling guilty.

4. The right to make mistakes and accept the responsibility for them.

5. The right to be listened to, and taken seriously.

6. The right to change one's mind.

7. The right to ask for what you want.

8. The right to put yourself first, sometimes.

9. The right to set one's own priorities.

10. The right to refuse justification for one's feelings or behavior.

FOUR BEHAVIORAL RESPONSE PATTERNS

Nonassertive Behavior

Assertive Behavior

Aggressive Behavior

Passive-Aggressive Behavior

CHAPTER 12: PSYCHOPHARMACOLOGY

CHAPTER FOCUS

The focus of this chapter is to introduce the student to the major drugs used in the psychiatric setting. Those presented include anxiolytics, antidepressants, antimanic agents, antipsychotics, antiparkinsonian agents, anticonvulsants, and sedative-hypnotics. The role of the nurse in administration of these medications and inpatient education is emphasized.

LEARNING OBJECTIVES

After reading this chapter, the student will be able to:

1. Discuss historical perspectives related to psychopharmacology.
2. Describe indications, actions, contraindications, and precautions of the following classifications of drugs:
   a. antianxiety agents
   b. antidepressants
   c. antimanics
   d. antipsychotics
   e. antiparkinsonian agents
   f. anticonvulsants
   g. sedative-hypnotics
3. Discuss common side effects and nursing implications for each classification, including patient/family education.

KEY TERMS

hypertensive crisis
priapism
retrograde ejaculation
gynecomastia
amenorrhea
agranulocytosis
extrapyramidal symptoms

akinesia
akathisia
dystonia
oculogyric crisis
tardive dyskinesia
neuroleptic malignant syndrome

CHAPTER OUTLINE/LECTURE NOTES

I.   Historical Perspectives
     A. Neuroleptics were introduced into the United States in the 1950's.
     B. Intended to be used as an adjunct to individual or group psychotherapy.
II. Antianxiety Agents
     A. Indications: anxiety disorders, anxiety symptoms, acute alcohol withdrawal, skeletal muscle spasms, convulsive disorders, status epilepticus and preoperative sedation and relief of anxiety.
     B. Actions: depression of the central nervous system.
     C. Contraindications/precautions: contraindicated in known hypersensitivity and in combination with other CNS depressants. Caution with elderly and debilitated patients.
     D. Chemical groups: antihistamines, benzodiazepines, metathiazanones, propanediols, miscellaneous.
     E. Side effects and nursing implications.
     F. Patient/family education.
III. Antidepressants
     A. Indications: dysthymic disorder; major depression; depression associated with organic disease, alcoholism, schizophrenia, or mental retardation; depressive phase of bipolar disorder; and depression accompanied by anxiety.

B. Action: block the reuptake of norepinephrine and serotonin by the neurons, thereby increasing their concentrations.

C. Contraindications/precautions: contraindicated in known hypersensitivity, acute phase of recovery from myocardial infarction, and in angle-closure glaucoma. Caution should be taken in prescribing for elderly, debilitated, or patients with hepatic, cardiac, or renal insufficiency. Caution also with psychotic patients, patients with benign prostatic hypertrophy, and those with history of seizures.

D. Chemical groups: unicyclic, bicyclic, tricyclics, tetracyclics, monoamine oxidase inhibitors, and others.

E. Side effects and nursing implications.

F. Patient/family education.

IV. Antimanics

A. Indications: prevention and treatment of manic episodes associated with bipolar disorder. Also used for depression associated with bipolar disorder.

B. Action: enhances the reuptake of norepinephrine and serotonin in the brain, lowering levels in the body and resulting in decreased hyperactivity.

C. Contraindications/precautions: contraindicated in known hypersensitivity, individuals with severe cardiovascular or renal disease, severe dehydration, sodium depletion, brain damage, and during pregnancy and lactation.

D. Chemical group: lithium carbonate.

E. Side effects and nursing implications.

F. Patient/family education.

V. Antipsychotics

A. Indications: treatment of acute and chronic psychoses. Selected agents are also used as antiemetics, in the treatment of intractable hiccoughs, and for the control of tics and vocal utterances in Tourette's disorder.

B. Action: unknown. Thought to block postsynaptic dopamine receptors in the basal ganglia, hypothalamus, limbic system, brainstem, and medulla.

C. Contraindications/precautions: contraindicated in known hypersensitivity and in lactation. Caution is advised with elderly and debilitated patients; those with hepatic, cardiac, or renal disease; and those who are pregnant. They should not be discontinued abruptly.

D. Chemical groups: long-acting barbiturates, hydantoins, benzodiazepines, and carbamazepine.

E. Side effects and nursing implications.

F. Patient/family education.

VIII. Sedative-Hypnotics

A. Indications: short-term management of various anxiety states and to treat insomnia.

B. Action: depression of the central nervous system.

C. Contraindications/precautions: contraindicated in known hypersensitivity. Caution advised with patients with hepatic dysfunction or severe renal impairment. Caution also advised with suicidal patients, and patients who have been addicted to drugs previously.

D. Chemical groups: barbiturates, benzodiazepines, miscellaneous.

E. Side effects and nursing implications.

F. Patient/family education.

IX. Summary

X. Review Questions

91

LEARNING ACTIVITIES

PSYCHOTROPIC MEDICATION QUIZ

Please fill in the blanks and answer the questions in the space provided:

1. What is the mechanism of action by which antidepressant medications achieve the desired effect (regardless of the different physiological processes by which this action is accomplished)?

2. For what must the nurse be on the alert with the patient who is receiving antidepressant medication?

3. As the nurse, when would you expect the patient to begin showing signs of symptomatic relief after the initiation of antidepressant therapy?

4. Name an example of a tricyclic antidepressant:_____.
    Name an example of a monamine oxydase inhibitor:_____.

5. Describe some common side effects and nursing implications for tricyclic antidepressants.

6. _____ is the most potentially life-threatening adverse effect of MAO inhibitors. Symptoms for which the nurse and patient must be on the alert include:_____. What must be done to prevent these symptoms from occurring? (Your answer must include some examples.)

7. Lithium carbonate is the drug of choice for _____. Many times when these individuals are started on lithium therapy, the physician also orders an antipsychotic medication. Why might he or she do this?

8. There is a narrow margin between the therapeutic and toxic serum levels of lithium carbonate. What is the therapeutic range, and list the initial signs and symptoms of lithium toxicity.

9. Describe some nursing implications for the patient on lithium therapy.

10. What is the mechanism of action for antianxiety medications?

11. What is the most commonly used group of antianxiety drugs? Give two examples.

12. What are the most common side effects of antianxiety drugs?

13. What must the patient on long term antianxiety therapy be instructed in order to prevent a potentially life-threatening situation?

14. What is the mechanism of action that produces the desired effect with antipsychotic medications (regardless of the physiological process by which this action is accomplished)?

15. Phenothiazines are the most commonly used antipsychotic group. Give two examples of phenothiazines.

16. Describe potential adverse hormonal effects associated with antipsychotic therapy.

17. Agranulocytosis is a relatively rare, but potentially very serious, side effect of antipsychotic therapy. The nurse and patient should be on the alert for symptoms of _____, _____, and _____.

18. Neuroleptic malignant syndrome (NMS) is also a rare, but potentially fatal, side effect of antipsychotic drugs. List symptoms for which the nurse must be on the alert when assessing for NMS.

19. Describe the symptoms of extrapyramidal side effects associated with antipsychotic therapy.

20. What is the classification of medication that is commonly prescribed for drug-induced extrapyramidal reactions? Give two examples of these medications.

ANTIANXIETY AGENTS

INDICATION:	Management of anxiety
ACTION:	CNS depression

COMMON GROUPS AND EXAMPLES:

Benzodiazepines:	Alprazolam (Xanax) Chlordiazepoxide (Librium) Diazepam (Valium)
Antihistamines:	Hydroxyzine (Atarax; Vistaril)
Miscellaneous:	Buspirone (BuSpar)

SIDE EFFECTS:	Drowsiness, confusion, tolerance (except with BuSpar)

ANTIDEPRESSANTS

INDICATION: Treatment of Depression

ACTION: Increase norepinephrine and serotonin

COMMON GROUPS AND
EXAMPLES:

    Unicyclic: Bupropion (Wellbutrin)
    Bicyclic: Fluoxetine (Prozac)
    Tricyclics: Amitriptyline (Elavil)
                Imipramine (Tofranil)
                Desipramine (Norpramin)
                Nortriptyline (Aventyl)
    Monoamine Oxidase
    Inhibitors: Phenelzine (Nardil)
                Isocarboxazid (Marplan)
    Other: Trazodone (Desyrel)

SIDE EFFECTS: Anticholinergic, sedation, orthostatic
                       hypotension, hypertensive crisis (MAOI's)

ANTIMANIC AGENTS

INDICATION: Prevention and treatment of manic episodes

ACTION: Decreases levels of serotonin and norepinephrine

DRUG OF CHOICE: **COMMON TRADE NAMES:**
Lithium Carbonate   Eskalith, Lithane, Lithobid, Carbolith, Lithizine, Lithotabs

SIDE EFFECTS: Dry mouth, GI upset, tremors, pulse irregularities, polyuria, weight gain

TOXICITY: Serum level should not go above 1.5. Initial symptoms of toxicity include: ataxia, blurred vision, persistent n/v, severe diarrhea, tinnitis.

ANTIPSYCHOTICS

INDICATION: Treatment of acute and chronic psychoses

ACTION: May decrease levels or block action of dopamine in the brain

COMMON GROUPS AND EXAMPLES:

Phenothiazines:	Chlorpromazine (Thorazine)
	Fluphenazine (Prolixin)
	Thioridazine (Mellaril)
Thioxanthenes:	Thiothixene (Navane)
Butyrophenone:	Haloperidol (Haldol)
Dibenzoxazepine:	Loxapine (Loxitane)
Dihydroindolone:	Molindone (Moban)
Dibenzodiazepine:	Clozapine (Clozaril)

SIDE EFFECTS: Anticholinergic, sedation, photosensitivity, hormonal effects, agranulocytosis, extrapyramidal symptoms, tardive dyskinesia, neuroleptic malignant syndrome

ANTIPARKINSONIAN AGENTS

INDICATIONS: Treatment of symptoms of parkinsonism

ACTION: Restores balance between acetylcholine and dopamine

COMMON GROUPS AND EXAMPLES:

Anticholinergics:	Benztropine (Cogentin)
	Procyclidine (Kemadrin)
	Trihexyphenidyl (Artane)
Antihistamines:	Diphenhydramine (Benadryl)
Dopaminergic Agonist:	Amantadine (Symmetrel)
	Bromocriptine (Parlodel)
	Levodopa (Dopar, Larodopa)

SIDE EFFECTS: Anticholinergic, GI upset, sedation, orthostatic hypotension, exacerbation of psychoses

ANTICONVULSANTS

INDICATION: Management of various types of seizure activity

ACTION: Most depress the central nervous system. Carbamazepine's action is unknown.

COMMON GROUPS AND EXAMPLES:

Long-acting barbituates: Phenobarbital (Luminal)
Primidone (Mysoline)

Hydantoins: Phenytoin (Dilantin)
Mephenytoin (Mesantoin)

Benzodiazepines: Clonazepam (Klonopin)
Clorazepate (Tranxene)
Diazepam (Valium)

Iminostilbene derivative: Carbamazepine (Tegretol)

SIDE EFFECTS: Sedation, decreased mental alertness, GI upset, liver damage, agranulocytosis, thrombocytopenia, gingival hyperplasia (hydantoins)

SEDATIVE-HYPNOTICS

INDICATION: Short-term management of anxiety or insomnia

ACTION: Depresses the central nervous system.

COMMON GROUPS AND EXAMPLES:

Barbiturates:	Phenobarbitol (Luminal)
	Secobarital (Seconal)
	Pentobarbital (Nembutal)
Benzodiazepines:	Flurazepam (Dalmane)
	Temazepam (Restoril)
	Triazolam (Halcion)
Miscellaneous:	Chloral hydrate (Noctec)
	Ethchlorvynol (Placidyl)

SIDE EFFECTS: Drowsiness, confusion, tolerance, "hangover" effect

CHAPTER 13: ELECTROCONVULSIVE THERAPY

CHAPTER FOCUS

The focus of this chapter is to introduce the student to the use of electroconvulsive therapy in psychiatry. The role of the nurse in the administration of electroconvulsive therapy is described.

LEARNING OBJECTIVES

After reading this chapter, the student will be able to:

1. Define electroconvulsive therapy (ECT).
2. Discuss historical perspectives related to electroconvulsive therapy.
3. Discuss indications, contraindications, mechanism of action, and side effects of electroconvulsive therapy.
4. Identify risks associated with electroconvulsive therapy.
5. Describe the role of the nurse in the administration of electroconvulsive therapy.

KEY TERMS

electroconvulsive therapy (ECT)   pharmacoconvulsive therapy
insulin coma therapy

CHAPTER OUTLINE/LECTURE NOTES

I.   Electroconvulsive Therapy (ECT) Defined
      A. ECT is the induction of a grand mal (generalized) seizure through the application of electrical current to the brain.
      B. Applied through electrodes placed bilaterally in the frontotemporal region, or unilaterally on the same side as the dominant hand.
      C. Amount of electrical current is determined by the type of machine being used, as well as the patient's condition. typical range: 70 to 125 volts for 0.7 to 1.5 seconds. Duration of the resulting seizure is 25 to 90 seconds.
      D. Most patients require an average of six to ten treatments, but some may not reach a maximal response until after 20 to 25 treatments.
      E. Usually administered every other day, for three times per week.
II.   Historical Perspectives
      A. The first treatment was performed in 1938 in Rome.
      B. Other types of somatic therapies had been tried prior to that time: insulin coma therapy and pharmacoconvulsive therapy.
      C. With insulin coma therapy, an injection of insulin produced a hypoglycemic coma, which was believed to alleviate the symptoms of schizophrenia. A number of fatalities occurred with insulin therapy, and it is very rarely used today.
      D. Pharmacoconvulsive therapy involved induction of convulsions with intramuscular injections of camphor in oil. The originator of this therapy believed this treatment also alleviated schizophrenic symptoms. he switched to the use of pentylenetetrazol when camphor was found to be unreliable. Some successes were reported in terms of reduction of psychotic symptoms, and this method was used until the advent of electroconvulsive therapy.
      E. Electroconvulsive therapy was widely accepted from around 1940 to 1955. This period was followed by a 20-year span during which ECT was considered objectionable by both the psychiatric profession and the lay public alike. A second peak of acceptance began around 1975 and has been increasing to the present.
      F. Approximately 60,000 to 100,000 people per year receive ECT treatments in the United States.

III. Indications
    A. Electroconvulsive therapy has been shown to be effective in the treatment of severe depression. It is usually not considered the treatment of choice for depression, but may be administered following a trial of therapy with antidepressant medication.
    B. ECT is also indicated in the treatment of manic episodes of bipolar affective disorder. It has been shown to be effective in treating manic patients who are refractory to lithium therapy.
    C. ECT can induce a remission in some patients who present with acute schizophrenia. It seems to be of little value in the treatment of chronic schizophrenia.

IV. Contraindications
    A. The only absolute contraindication for ECT is increased intracranial pressure (from brain tumor, recent CVA, or other cerebrovascular lesion).
    B. Individuals at high risk with electroconvulsive therapy include those with myocardial infarction or cerebrovascular accident within the preceding three months, aortic or cerebral aneurysm, severe underlying hypertension, and congestive heart failure.

V. Mechanism of Action
    A. The exact mechanism of action by which electroconvulsive therapy effects a therapeutic response is unknown. Some credibility has been given to the biochemical theory that ECT results in significant increases in the circulating levels of serotonin, norepinephrine, and dopamine.

VI. Side Effects
    A. Most common side effects: temporary memory loss and confusion.

VII. Risks Associated with Electroconvulsive Therapy
    A. Mortality
        1. Mortality rate from ECT falls somewhere in the range between 0.01% and 0.04%. Although death is rare, when it does occur, it is usually related to cardiovascular complications.
    B. Permanent memory loss
        1. Studies have shown that a small subgroup of patients receiving ECT may suffer permanent memory impairment.
    C. Brain damage
        1. Critics of ECT remain adamant in their belief that the procedure always results in some degree of immediate brain damage. There are, however, no current data to substantiate that ECT produces any permanent changes in brain structure or functioning.

VIII. Role of the Nurse in Electroconvulsive Therapy
    A. The nursing process is the method of delivery of care for the patient receiving electroconvulsive therapy.
    B. The patient must receive a thorough physical exam prior to initiation of therapy. This exam should include assessment of cardiovascular and pulmonary status, as well as laboratory blood and urine studies. A skeletal history and x-ray assessment should also be considered.
    C. The nurse must ensure that informed consent has been granted. The nurse must also assess mood, level of anxiety, thought and communication patterns, and vital signs. Appropriate nursing diagnoses are formulated based on assessment data.
    D. Nurses prepare the patient for the treatment by having him or her void, removing dentures, eyeglasses or contact lenses, jewelry, and hairpins. Atropine sulfate or glycopyrrolate is administered according to physician's orders approximately 30 minutes prior to the treatment.
    E. In the treatment room, the anesthesiologist administers a muscle relaxant (usually succinylcholine) and a short-acting anesthetic (such as thiopental sodium or methohexital sodium). The patient receives oxygen prior to the treatment.
    F. An airway/bite block is used to facilitate the patient's airway patency. Electrodes are placed on the temples to deliver the electrical stimulation.
    G. The nurse assists the psychiatrist and the anesthesiologist as required, as well as providing support to the patient, both physically and emotionally.
    H. Following the treatment, the nurse remains with the patient until he or she is fully awake. Vital signs are taken every 15 minutes for the first hour. The patient is oriented to time and place, and given an explanation of what has occurred.
    I. Evaluation of changes in patient behavior are made to determine improvement and provide assistance in deciding the number of treatments that will be administered.

IX. Summary

X. Review Questions

LEARNING ACTIVITY

ELECTROCONVULSIVE THERAPY

Match the terms on the left with the descriptions listed on the right.

_____ 1. atropine sulfate

_____ 2. succinylcholine

_____ 3. thiopental sodium

_____ 4. increased intracranial pressure

_____ 5. temporary memory loss and confusion

_____ 6. major depression

_____ 7. oxygen

_____ 8. informed consent

_____ 9. norepinephrine and serotonin

_____ 10. recent myocardial infarction

a. major indication for ECT

b. the only absolute contraindication for ECT

c. given prior to ECT to decrease secretions and increase heart rate

d. administered prior to, during and following ECT

e. most common cause of mortality associated with ECT

f. administered as a short-acting anesthetic

g. thought to be increased by ECT

h. most common side effects of ECT

i. required before treatment can be initiated

j. muscle relaxant given to prevent bone fractures

ELECTROCONVULSIVE THERAPY

INDICATION:	Major Depression Mania Acute Schizophrenia
ACTION:	Unknown. Thought to increase levels of norepinephrine and serotonin in the brain.
CONTRAINDICATION:	Increased intracranial pressure.
HIGH RISK FOR ECT:	Recent MI or CVA, aneurysm, severe hypertension, CHF.
SIDE EFFECTS:	Temporary memory loss and confusion.
RISKS:	Mortality, permanent memory loss, brain damage.

CHAPTER 14: BEHAVIOR THERAPY

CHAPTER FOCUS

The focus of this chapter is on various concepts associated with learning, and on techniques for modification of learned behaviors. The role of the nurse in behavior therapy is emphasized.

LEARNING OBJECTIVES

After reading this chapter, the student will be able to:

1. Discuss the principles of classical and operant conditioning as foundations for behavior therapy.
2. Identify various techniques used in the modification of patient behavior.
3. Implement the principles of behavior therapy utilizing the steps of the nursing process.

KEY TERMS

classical conditioning	shaping
unconditioned response	modeling
conditioned response	Premack principle
unconditioned stimulus	extinction
conditioned stimulus	flooding
stimulus generalization	token economy
operant conditioning	time out
positive reinforcement	reciprocal inhibition
negative reinforcement	overt sensitization
aversive stimulus	covert sensitization
discriminative stimulus	systematic desensitization
contingency contracting	

CHAPTER OUTLINE/LECTURE NOTES

I. Introduction
   A. A behavior is considered to be maladaptive when it:
      1. is age-inappropriate
      2. interferes with adaptive functioning
      3. is misunderstood by others in terms of cultural inappropriateness
   B. The behavioral approach to therapy is that people have become what they are through learning processes, or through the interaction of the environment with their genetic endowment.
   C. The basic assumption is that problematic behaviors occur when there has been inadequate learning, and therefore can be corrected through the provision of appropriate learning experiences.
II. Classical Conditioning
   A. Introduced by Russian physiologist Pavlov in his experiments with dogs.
   B. Pavlov related that the dogs salivated when presented with food (unconditioned response).
   C. Soon learned that dogs salivated when food came into view (conditioned response).
   D. He introduced an unrelated stimulus (the sound of a bell) with presentation of food.
   E. He learned that the dogs soon began salivating (conditioned response) at the sound of the bell alone (conditioned stimulus).
   F. When a similar response is elicited from similar stimuli, it is called stimulus generalization.
III. Operant Conditioning
   A. Introduced by American psychologist B. F. Skinner.

B. Basic assumption: that the connection between a stimulus and a response is strengthened or weakened by the consequences of the response.

C. A stimulus that follows a behavior (or response) is called a reinforcer.

D. When the reinforcing stimulus increases the probability that the behavior will reoccur, it is called a positive reinforcer.

E. When the reinforcing stimulus increases the probability that a behavior will reoccur by removal of an undesirable reinforcing stimulus, it is called a negative reinforcer.

F. A stimulus that follows a behavioral response and decreases the probability that the behavior will reoccur is called an aversive stimulus or punisher.

IV. Techniques for Modifying Patient Behavior

A. Shaping. In shaping the behavior of another, reinforcements are given for increasingly closer approximations to the desired response.

B. Modeling. Modeling refers to the learning of new behaviors by imitating the behavior of others.

C. Premack principle. This principle states that a frequently-occurring response can serve as a positive reinforcement for a response.

D. Extinction. The gradual decrease in frequency or disappearance of a response when the positive reinforcement is withheld.

E. Contingency Contracting. A contract for behavioral change is developed. Positive and negative reinforcers for performing the desired behaviors, as well as aversive reinforcers for failure to perform, are stated explicitly in the contract.

F. Token economy. A type of contingency contracting in which the reinforcers for desired behaviors are presented in the form of tokens. The tokens may then be exchanged for designated privileges.

G. Time out. An aversive stimulus or punishment during which the patient is removed from the environment where the unacceptable behavior is being exhibited. The patient is usually isolated so that reinforcement from the attention of others is absent.

H. Reciprocal Inhibition. Also called counterconditioning, this technique serves to decrease or eliminate a behavior by introducing a more adaptive behavior, but one that is incompatible with the unacceptable behavior.

I. Overt sensitization. An aversion therapy that produces unpleasant consequences for undesirable behavior.

J. Covert sensitization. This aversion technique relies on the individual's imagination to produce unpleasant symptoms as consequences for undesirable behavior.

K. Systematic desensitization. A technique to assist individuals to overcome their fear of a phobic stimulus. A systematic hierarchy of events associated with the phobic stimulus is used to gradually desensitize the individual.

L. Flooding. Sometimes called implosive therapy, this technique is used to desensitize individuals to phobic stimuli. It differs from systematic desensitization in that, instead of working up a hierarchy of anxiety producing stimuli, the individual is "flooded" with a continuous presentation of the phobic stimulus until it no longer elicits anxiety.

V. Role of the Nurse in Behavior Therapy

A. The nursing process is the vehicle for delivery of nursing care with patients requiring assistance with behavior modification.

B. Assessment of behaviors that are unacceptable for age and cultural inappropriateness is conducted.

C. Nursing diagnoses are formulated and outcome criteria are established.

D. A plan for behavior modification is devised utilizing techniques thought to be most appropriate for the patient.

E. All members of the treatment team must be made aware of the behavior modification plan. Consistency among all staff is required for implementation to be successful.

F. Evaluation of care is based upon achievement of the outcome criteria.

VI. Summary

VII. Review Questions

LEARNING ACTIVITY

TECHNIQUES FOR MODIFYING PATIENT BEHAVIOR

Match the techniques listed on the left to the situations described on the right.

_____ 1. Shaping

_____ 2. Modeling

_____ 3. Premack Principle

_____ 4. Extinction

_____ 5. Contingency Contracting

_____ 6. Token Economy

_____ 7. Time Out

_____ 8. Reciprocal Inhibition

_____ 9. Overt Sensitization

_____ 10. Covert Sensitization

_____ 11. Systematic Desensitization

_____ 12. Flooding

a. John had tried many times without success to stop drinking. His physician has suggested trying disulfiram therapy, and John has agree.

b. Two-year-old Missy has had temper tantrums for six months. They have become progressively worse, as her Mother always gives in and lets Missy have what she wants in order to end the tantrum. The therapist suggested that Mom turn and walk away when a tantrum occurs.

c. The therapist is trying to teach 3-year-old Billy to use sign language. She rewards hi when he watches her sign; then rewards him when he attempts to sign sign himself; and finally only rewards him when he signs correctly.

d. Nancy has a phobia of flying. The therapist asks Nancy to mentally imagine, as she is confronted with a continuous presentation of stimuli associated with flying, until she no longer feels anxious by the images elicited.

e. Eleven-year-old Timmy likes to bully the younger kids. He refuses to do anything his parents ask, and talks back to the teachers when they give him direction. The therapist outlines for Timmy which behaviors are acceptable and which are not. She explains to Timmy that he will receive a "chip" each time he behaves appropriately, and he may use the chips to buy certain privileges.

f. Ten-year-old Sonja begged her Mother to let her take piano lessons. Her Mother agreed, but now Sonja wants to watch TV all the time instead of practicing her piano lesson. Her Mother tells Sonja she can only watch TV after she has practiced her piano lesson.

g. Thirteen-year-old Lisa is a patient on the adolescent psychiatric unit. Each time she is with a group of her peers she begins using offensive, vulgar language. Her peers provide positive reinforcement by laughing at her. The therapist tells Lisa that each time this occurs she will spend time alone in the isolation room.

h. Janet, age 25, has been obese since childhood. The therapist is helping Janet in her effort to lose weight. The therapist teaches Janet to visualize in her mind foods that are offensive to her and that make her feel nauseated. Each time Janet is tempted to eat more than her reducing diet allows, she is to conjure up this image in her mind.

i. Angie has been in trouble with her parents and school authorities for inappropriate behavior. Angie strongly admires her Aunt Sylvia, her mother's sister, who is a successful newspaper reporter in a nearby city. Angie is sent to live with her aunt in hopes that she will imitate her cherished aunt's behavior and life style.

j. Sixteen-year-old Andy loses his temper at the slightest provocation on the adolescent psychiatric unit. The therapist draws up a written contract with Andy. Rewards for managing his anger are explicitly stated, as are punishments for losing his temper.

k. Sandy experiences test anxiety. She becomes overwhelmed with anxiety each time she is faced with an exam. The therapist teaches Sandy to perform relaxation exercises before, and sometimes even during, an exam when she feels anxiety escalating.

l. Barbara has an extreme fear of dogs. She panics when she sees one. The therapist attempts to help Barbara overcome her fear by exposing her to a step-by-step process in which she gradually is able to look at a dog, touch one, and be in the presence of one without experiencing panic anxiety.

CLASSICAL CONDITIONING

Unconditioned Stimulus

Unconditioned Response

Conditioned Stimulus

Conditioned Response

Stimulus Generalization

OPERANT CONDITIONING

Stimulus

Positive Reinforcement

Negative Reinforcement

Aversive Stimulus
(Punishment)

Discriminative Stimuli

TECHNIQUES FOR BEHAVIOR MODIFICATION

Shaping

Modeling

Premack Principle

Extinction

Contingency Contracting

Token Economy

Time Out

Reciprocal Inhibition

Overt Sensitization

Covert Sensitization

Systematic Desensitization

Flooding

CHAPTER 15: DISORDERS USUALLY FIRST EVIDENT IN INFANCY, CHILDHOOD OR ADOLESCENCE

CHAPTER FOCUS

The focus of this chapter is on psychiatric disorders usually first evident in infancy, childhood, or adolescence. Symptomatology and predisposing factors are described. Role of the nurse in care of these patients is emphasized.

LEARNING OBJECTIVES

After reading this chapter, the student will be able to:

1. Identify psychiatric disorders usually first evident in infancy, childhood, or adolescence.
2. Discuss predisposing factors implicated in the etiology of mental retardation, autistic disorder, behavior disorders, anxiety disorders of childhood/adolescence, eating disorders, and gender identity disorders.
3. Identify symptomatology and utilize the information in the assessment of patients with the above disorders.
4. Identify nursing diagnoses common to patients with these disorders and select appropriate nursing interventions for each.
5. Discuss relevant criteria for evaluating nursing care of patients with selected infant, childhood, and adolescent psychiatric disorders.
6. Describe various treatment modalities relevant to care of patients with these disorders.

KEY TERMS

aggression   clinging
autism   amenorrhea
temperament   binge and purge
impulsiveness   body image
negativism   gender

CHAPTER OUTLINE/LECTURE NOTES

I.   Introduction
     A. It is often difficult to determine if a child's behavior is indicative of emotional problems
     B. The DSM-III-R suggests that an emotional problem exists if the behavioral manifestations:
        1. are not age appropriate
        2. deviate from cultural norms
        3. create deficits or impairments in adaptive functioning
II. Developmental Disorders
     A. Mental retardation (MR)
        1. Defined by deficits in general intellectual functioning (as measured by intelligence quotient exams) and adaptive functioning (the ability to adapt to the requirements of daily living and the expectations of age and cultural group).
        2. Predisposing factors
           a. Heredity factors
              (1) Implicated in approximately 5% of the cases.
              (2) Include:
                 (a) inborn errors of metabolism, such as Tay-Sachs disease, phenylketonuria, and hyperglycemia.
                 (b) chromosomal disorders, such as Down's syndrome and Klinefelter's syndrome.
                 (c) single gene abnormalities, such as tuberous sclerosis and neurofibromatosis.

      b. Prenatal factors
        (1) Account for 30% of MR cases.
        (2) Damages may occur in response to:
          (a) toxicity associated with maternal ingestion of alcohol or other drugs.
          (b) maternal illnesses and infections during pregnancy.
          (c) complications of pregnancy, such as toxemia and uncontrolled diabetes.
      c. Perinatal factors
        (1) Account for approximately 10% of cases of MR.
        (2) Can be caused by:
          (a) trauma or complications of the birth process that result in deprivation of oxygen to the infant.
          (b) premature birth.
      d. Postnatal factors
        (1) Account for approximately 5% of cases of MR.
        (2) Can be caused by:
          (a) infections, such as meningitis and encephalitis.
          (b) poisonings, such as from insecticides, medications, lead.
          (c) physical traumas, such as head injuries, asphyxiation, and hyperpyrexia.
      e. Social, cultural, and environmental factors
        (1) Account for approximately 20% of cases of MR.
        (2) May be attributed to:
          (a) deprivation of nurturance and social stimulation.
          (b) nutritional deficiencies.
   3. Application of the nursing process
      a. Degree of severity of mental retardation is identified by level of intelligence quotient.
      b. Four levels have been delineated: mild, moderate, severe, and profound.
      c. Nurses must assess strengths as well as limitations in order to encourage the patient to be as independent as possible.
      d. It is important to include family members in the planning and implementation of care.
      e. Family members should receive information regarding the scope of the condition, realistic expectations and patient potentials, methods for modifying behavior as required, community resources from whom they may seek assistance and support.
      f. Evaluation of care given to the mentally retarded patient should reflect positive behavioral change.
  B. Autistic disorder
    1. Characterized by a withdrawal of the child into the self and into a fantasy world of his or her own creation.
    2. The disorder is rare and may occur in infancy (before age 36 months) or childhood (after age 36 months).
    3. Predisposing factors
      a. Social environment. Causative factors are thought to include parental rejection, child responses to deviant parental personality characteristics, family breakup, family stress, insufficient stimulation, and faulty communication patterns.
      b. Biological factors.
        (1) Genetics. Sibling and twin studies have revealed a strong evidence that genetic factors play a significant role.
        (2) Neurological factors. Conditions that cause brain dysfunction have been implicated:
          (a) maternal rubella, untreated phenylketonuria, tuberous sclerosis, anoxia during birth, encephalitis, infantile spasms, and fragile X syndrome.
          (b) other diseases and syndromes that affect the CNS have also been implicated: mental retardation, congenital syphilis, epilepsy and congenital rubella.
    4. Application of the nursing process
      a. Symptomatology
        (1) Impairment in social interaction.
        (2) Impairment in communication and imaginative activity.
        (3) Restricted activities and interests.
      b. Nursing intervention is aimed at protection of the child from self-directed violence, and improvement in social functioning, verbal communication, and personal identity.
III. Disruptive Behavior Disorders
  A. Attention-Deficit Hyperactivity Disorder (ADHD)
    1. Essential features include developmentally inappropriate degrees of inattention, impulsiveness, and hyperactivity.

113

2. Predisposing factors
   a. Biological influences
      (1) Genetics. Frequency among family members has been noted.
      (2) Biochemical theory. Implicates a deficit of dopamine and norepinephrine in the brain.
      (3) Pre-, peri-, and post-natal factors
         (a) prenatal factors include maternal smoking during pregnancy.
         (b) perinatal factors include prematurity, signs of fetal distress, prolonged labor, and perinatal asphyxia.
         (c) Postnatal factors include cerebral palsy, epilepsy, and CNS trauma or infections.
   b. Environmental influences
      (1) Environmental lead.
      (2) Diet factors, including food dyes and additives, and sugar.
   c. Psychosocial influences
      (1) Disorganized or chaotic environments.
      (2) Child abuse or neglect.
      (3) Family history of alcoholism, hysterical or sociopathic behaviors.
      (4) Developmental learning disorders.
3. Application of the nursing process
   a. Symptomatology
      (1) Highly distractible with extremely limited attention span.
      (2) Difficulty forming satisfactory interpersonal relationships.
      (3) Low frustration tolerance and outbursts of temper.
      (4) Excessive levels of activity, restlessness, and fidgeting.
   b. Nursing intervention is aimed at protection from injury due to excessive hyperactivity, improvement in social interaction, self-esteem, and compliance with task expectations.
4. Psychopharmacological intervention
   a. Drug of choice: central nervous system stimulants.
   b. Examples: dextroamphetamine, methylphenidate, and pemoline.
   c. Effects on children with ADHD: increased attention span, control of hyperactive behavior, and improvement in learning ability.
   d. Side effects: insomnia, anorexia, weight loss, tachycardia, and temporary decrease in rate of growth and development. Tolerance can occur.
   e. A drug "holiday" should be attempted periodically under direction of the physician to determine effectiveness of the medication and need for continuation.

B. Conduct disorder
   1. A persistent pattern of conduct in which the basic rights of others and major age-appropriate societal norms or rules are violated. Three types: group, solitary aggressive, and undifferentiated.
   2. Predisposing factors
      a. Biological influences
         (1) Genetics. Twins and non-twin sibling studies indicate a higher incidence among those who have family members with the disorder.
         (2) Temperament. Children who are born with "difficult" temperaments were found to have a significantly higher degree of aggressive behavior later in life.
         (3) Biochemical. Elevated levels of plasma testosterone have been correlated with aggressive behavior.
      b. Psychosocial influences
         (1) Impaired social-cognition. Rejection by peers may predispose to aggressive behavior.
      c. Family influences
         (1) The following family dynamics may contribute development of conduct disorders;
            (a) parental rejection
            (b) inconsistent management with harsh discipline
            (c) early institutional living
            (d) frequent shifting of parental figures
            (e) large family size
            (f) absent father
            (g) parents with antisocial personality disorder or alcohol dependence
            (h) association with a delinquent subgroup
            (i) marital conflict and divorce
            (j) inadequate communication patterns

(k) parental permissiveness
3. Application of the nursing process
   a. Symptomatology
      (1) Physical aggression in the violation of the rights of others.
      (2) Use of drugs and alcohol.
      (3) Sexual permissiveness.
      (4) Use of projection as a defense mechanism.
      (5) Low self-esteem manifested by "tough-guy" image.
      (6) Inability to control anger.
      (7) Low academic achievement.
   b. Nursing intervention is aimed at protection of others from patient's physical aggression; improvement in social interaction and self-esteem; and acceptance of responsibility for own behavior.
C. Oppositional Defiant Disorder (ODD)
1. Characterized by negativistic, hostile, and defiant behavior (more severe than seen in most people of the same mental age).
2. Predisposing factors
   a. Biological influences. Role not established.
   b. Family influences. If power and control are issues for parents, or if they exercise authority for their own needs, a power struggle can be established between the parents and the child that sets the stage for the development of ODD.
3. Application of the nursing process
   a. Symptomatology
      (1) Symptoms include passive-aggression exhibited by obstinacy, procrastination, disobedience, carelessness, negativism, dawdling, provocation, resistance to change, violation of minor rules, blocking out communications from others, and resistance to authority.
      (2) Other symptoms may include enuresis, encopresis, elective mutism, running away, school avoidance, school underachievement, eating and sleeping problems, temper tantrums, fighting, and argumentativeness.
      (3) Interpersonal relationships are impaired and school performance if often unsatisfactory.
   b. Nursing intervention is aimed at compliance with therapy, acceptance of responsibility for own behavior, increase in self-esteem, and improvement in social interaction.
IV. Anxiety Disorders of Childhood or Adolescence
A. Predominant clinical feature is anxiety. Three categories include:
1. Separation Anxiety Disorder
2. Avoidant Disorder of Childhood or Adolescence
3. Overanxious Disorder
B. Predisposing factors
1. Biological influences
   a. Genetics. Studies show that a greater number of children with relatives who manifest anxiety problems develop anxiety disorders themselves than do children with no such family patterns.
   b. Temperament. It is believed that certain individuals inherit a "disposition" toward developing anxiety disorders.
2. Environmental influences
   a. Stressful life events. It is thought that children who are already predisposed to developing anxiety disorders may be affected significantly by stressful life events.
3. Family influences
   a. Possible overattachment to the mother.
   b. Separation conflicts between parent and child.
   c. Families that are very close-knit and caring (separation anxiety).
   d. Most common in eldest children, small families, upper socioeconomic groups, and in families in which there is a concern about achievement (overanxious disorder).
   e. Overprotection by parents.
   f. Transfer of fears and anxieties from parents to child through role modeling.
C. Application of the nursing process
1. Symptomatology
   a. Separation Anxiety Disorder
      (1) Child has difficulty separating from mother.
      (2) Separation results in tantrums, crying, screaming, complaints of physical problems, and "clinging"

behaviors.
- (3) School reluctance or refusal.
- (4) Fear of harm to self or attachment figure.
- (5) Depressed mood is common.
  - b. Avoidant Disorder of Childhood or Adolescence
    - (1) Excessive and irrational fear of being around unfamiliar people.
    - (2) Non-assertiveness and lack of self-confidence are common.
    - (3) Severe impairment of social functioning.
    - (4) In adolescence, inhibition of normal psychosexual activity is common.
    - (5) Social isolation and depression.
  - c. Overanxious Disorder
    - (1) Unrealistic worrying about future events and about the appropriateness of their behavior in the past.
    - (2) Excessive concern about competence.
    - (3) Perfectionistic with desire to excel.
    - (4) Somatic complaints are common.
    - (5) Lack of self-confidence.
    - (6) Symptoms may be chronic and persist into adulthood.
  2. Nursing intervention is aimed at maintaining anxiety at moderate level or below; improvement in social interaction; and development of adaptive coping strategies that prevent maladaptive symptoms of anxiety in response to stressful situations.

V. Eating Disorders
  A. Characterized by gross disturbances in eating behavior.
  B. Predisposing factors
    1. Biological influences
      a. Genetics. A hereditary predisposition to eating disorders has been hypothesized on the basis of family histories and an apparent association with other disorders for which the likelihood of genetic influences exist.
      b. Neuroendocrine abnormalities. Some possibility of a primary hypothalamic dysfunction in anorexia nervosa. Also possible include elevated cerebral spinal fluid cortisol levels and impairment of dopaminergic regulation.
    2. Psychodynamic influences
      a. Suggest that eating disorders are the result of very early and profound disturbances in mother-infant interactions, resulting in retarded ego development and unfulfilled sense of separation-individuation.
    3. Family influences
      a. Conflict avoidance. Suggests that eating disorder serves to avoid conflict in the spousal relationship. Attention is refocused on the person with physical problem and away from marital conflict.
      b. Elements of power and control. Family may include passive father, domineering mother, and an overly dependent child. High value placed on perfectionism. Ambivalent feelings toward parents develop. Dysfunctional eating behaviors viewed as rebellion against the parents in a struggle for power and control.
  C. Application of the nursing process
    1. Symptomatology
      a. Anorexia nervosa
        (1) Morbid fear of obesity.
        (2) Gross distortion of body image.
        (3) Preoccupation with food, but refusal to eat.
        (4) Self-induced vomiting and/or abuse of laxatives or diuretics.
        (5) Loss of at least 15% of total body weight.
        (6) Amenorrhea.
        (7) Delayed psychosexual development.
        (8) Depression and anxiety common.
      b. Bulimia nervosa
        (1) Uncontrolled, rapid ingestion of large quantities of food over a short period of time (binging), followed by episodes of self-induced vomiting (purging).
        (2) Self-degradation and depressed mood usually follow a binge.
        (3) Abuse of laxatives or diuretics.
        (4) Weight is maintained close to normal.

          (5) Excessive vomiting and laxative/diuretic abuse may lead to problems with dehydration and electrolyte imbalance.

    2. Nursing intervention is aimed at restoration of nutrition and hydration; development of more adaptive coping mechanisms; and improvement in body image and self-esteem.

  D. Treatment modalities for eating disorders

    1. Behavior modification.

    2. Family therapy.

    3. Psychopharmacology.

VI. Gender Identity Disorders

  A. Occur when there is an incongruence between anatomic sex and gender identity. Three categories:

    1. Gender identity disorder of childhood.

    2. Transsexualism.

    3. Gender identity disorder of adolescence or adulthood.

  B. Predisposing factors

    1. Biological influences

      a. Little biological evidence exists to explain the etiology of gender identity disorders.

    2. Family influences

      a. Strong interests in opposite-gender activities and weak reinforcement of normative gender-role behavior by the parents.

      b. In boys, absence of a father, and encouragement of extreme physical and psychological closeness with the mother.

  C. Application of the nursing process

    1. Symptomatology

      a. Gender identity disorder of childhood

        (1) Profound disturbance in sense of masculinity or femininity.

        (2) Child insists he or she is of the opposite sex.

        (3) Aversion to physical characteristics of the biological sex.

        (4) Preoccupation with opposite sex stereotypic activities and dress.

        (5) Impairment of interpersonal functioning.

      b. Transsexualism

        (1) A person who has reached puberty and experiences persistent discomfort and a sense of inappropriateness about his or her anatomic sex.

        (2) May live as an individual of the opposite sex.

        (3) Desires hormonal therapy or surgery to generate a sex reassignment.

      c. Gender identity disorder of adolescence or adulthood, nontranssexual type

        (1) Persistent discomfort with assigned sex.

        (2) Cross-dressing.

        (3) May evolve into transsexualism.

    2. Nursing intervention for the patient with gender identity disorder of childhood is aimed at behaviors that are appropriate and culturally-acceptable for assigned sex, and improvement in social interaction and self-esteem.

VII. Summary

VIII. Review Questions

LEARNING ACTIVITY

DISORDERS OF INFANCY, CHILDHOOD, OR ADOLESCENCE

Match the disorders listed on the left to the behaviors associated with each on the right.

_____ 1. Mental Retardation

_____ 2. Autistic Disorder

_____ 3. Attention-Deficit Hyperactivity Disorder

_____ 4. Conduct Disorder

_____ 5. Oppositional Defiant Disorder

_____ 6. Separation Anxiety Disorder

_____ 7. Avoidant Disorder of Childhood or Adolescence

_____ 8. Overanxious Disorder

_____ 9. Anorexia Nervosa

_____ 10. Bulimia Nervosa

_____ 11. Gender Identity Disorder of Childhood

_____ 12. Transsexualism

_____ 13. Gender Identify Disorder of Adolescence or Adulthood

a. Binges and purges; self-degradation and depressed mood.

b. Violates the rights of others and societal norms and rules. Physical aggression and inability to control anger.

c. Identified by level of intelligence quotient and ability to perform at level expected for age and culture.

d. Screams and throws temper tantrums at anticipated separation from mother. Fear of harm to self or mother.

e. Cross-dressing and persistent discomfort with assigned sex in one who has reached puberty.

f. Unrealistic worrying about future events and about appropriateness of past behavior. Excessive concern about competence.

g. Child insists he or she is member of the opposite sex. Preoccupation with opposite sex stereotypic activities.

h. Withdrawal of the child into the self and into a fantasy world of his or her own creation.

i. Desires hormonal therapy or surgery to generate a sex reassignment.

j. Excessive and irrational fear of being around unfamiliar people.

k. Negativistic and defiant behavior, including obstinacy, procrastination, disobedience, resistance to change and authority.

l. Developmentally inappropriate degrees of inattention, impulsiveness, and hyperactivity.

m. Distorted body image; loss of 15% or more of ideal body weight; morbid fear of obesity; amenorrhea.

COMMON NURSING DIAGNOSES FOR DEVELOPMENTAL DISORDERS

MENTAL RETARDATION

Potential for Injury
Self-Care Deficit
Impaired Verbal Communication
Impaired Social Interaction

AUTISTIC DISORDER

Potential for Self-Mutilation
Impaired Social Interaction
Impaired Verbal Communication
Personal Identity Disturbance

COMMON NURSING DIAGNOSES FOR DISRUPTIVE BEHAVIOR DISORDERS

ATTENTION DEFICIT-HYPERACTIVITY DISORDER

Potential for Injury
Impaired Social Interaction
Self-Esteem Disturbance
Noncompliance (with task expectations)

CONDUCT DISORDER

Potential for Violence (directed toward others)
Impaired Social Interaction
Defensive Coping
Self-Esteem Disturbance

OPPOSITIONAL DEFIANT DISORDER

Noncompliance (with therapy)
Defensive Coping
Self-Esteem Disturbance
Impaired Social Interaction

COMMON NURSING DIAGNOSES FOR ANXIETY DISORDERS OF CHILDHOOD OR ADOLESCENCE

Anxiety (severe)

Ineffective Individual Coping

Impaired Social Interaction

COMMON NURSING DIAGNOSES FOR EATING DISORDERS

Altered Nutrition: Less than Body Requirements

Fluid Volume Deficit (actual or potential)

Ineffective Denial

Body Image Disturbance

Self-Esteem Disturbance

COMMON NURSING DIAGNOSES FOR GENDER IDENTITY DISORDER OF CHILDHOOD

Personal Identity Disturbance

Impaired Social Interaction

Self-Esteem Disturbance

CHAPTER 16: ORGANIC MENTAL SYNDROMES AND DISORDERS

CHAPTER FOCUS

The focus of this chapter is on individuals with organic mental syndromes and disorders. Predisposing factors and symptomatology are described, and the role of the nurse in caring for patients with these disorders is emphasized.

LEARNING OBJECTIVES

After reading this chapter, the student will be able to:

1. Describe various organic mental syndromes and disorders.
2. Discuss predisposing factors implicated in the etiology of organic mental syndromes and disorders.
3. Identify symptomatology and use the information in the assessment of patients with organic mental syndromes and disorders.
4. Identify nursing diagnoses common to patients with organic mental syndromes and disorders and select appropriate nursing interventions for each.
5. Discuss relevant criteria for evaluating nursing care of patients with organic mental syndromes and disorders.
6. Describe various treatment modalities relevant to care of patients with organic mental syndromes and disorders.

KEY TERMS

amphetamines	dementia
aphasia	opioids
apraxia	phencyclidine
cannabis	presenile
delirium	senile

CHAPTER OUTLINE/LECTURE NOTES

I.   Introduction
     A. These disorders represent the dysfunction, and in some instances the eventual loss, of mental functions in an otherwise alert and awake individual.
     B. The numbers of individuals with these disorders is growing because more people now survive into the high-risk period for dementia, which can strike at any time from middle age onward.
II. Syndrome vs. Disorder
     A. A syndrome refers to a cluster of signs and symptoms for which there is no known etiology (e.g., dementia, delirium).
     B. Disorders designate particular syndromes for which the etiology is known or presumed (e.g., multi-infarct dementia, alcohol withdrawal delirium).
     C. Organic mental syndromes and disorders may be chronic or acute, reversible or irreversible.
III. Organic Mental Syndromes
     A. Identified solely on the behavioral manifestations.
     B. If etiology is identified, syndrome is recategorized as a disorder.
     C. The DSM-III-R identifies 10 categories of syndromes:
         1. Delirium. The individual is extremely distractable, thinking is disorganized, speech is rambling and pressured. Disorientation and memory loss are evident. Level of consciousness is affected. Psychomotor activity may be agitated or vegetative. Emotions are labile. Autonomic manifestations are common. Onset is usually acute, and duration is usually brief.

2. Dementia. Impairment in memory, abstract thinking, judgment, and impulse control. Personal appearance and hygiene are often neglected. Language may not be affected, or aphasia may be present. Personality changes are common. The course is progressive and irreversible. The person eventually becomes totally dependent on others for daily care.

3. Amnestic syndrome. Impairment in short- and long-term memory. Disorientation and confabulation are common. Differs from dementia in that there is no impairment in abstract thinking or judgment, no other disturbances or higher cortical function, and no personality change.

4. Organic hallucinosis. Presence of persistent or recurrent hallucinations attributed to a specific organic factor.

5. Organic delusional syndrome. Presence of prominent delusions that can be attributed to a specific organic factor. Mild cognitive impairment may be evident, with disorientation and incoherent or rambling speech.

6. Organic mood syndrome. Persistent depression or elevation of mood that can be attributed to a specific organic factor.

7. Organic anxiety syndrome. Prominent, recurrent, panic attacks or generalized anxiety attributed to a specific organic factor.

8. Organic personality syndrome. A persistent personality disturbance attributable to a specific organic factor. The disturbance may represent a lifelong pattern of behavior or a change or accentuation of a previous personality trait.

9. Intoxication. A syndrome of symptoms that can be attributed to recent ingestion of a psychoactive substance that results in maladaptive behavioral changes. Type of symptoms depends upon the substance ingested, and may include any of the following:
   a. Alcohol
   b. Amphetamines
   c. Caffeine
   d. Cannabis
   e. Cocaine
   f. Inhalants
   g. Opioids
   h. Phencyclidine
   i. CNS depressants

10. Withdrawal. The development of a substance-specific syndrome that follows the cessation of, or reduction in, intake of a psychoactive substance that the person previously used regularly. Withdrawal disorders may be attributed to:
   a. Alcohol
   b. Amphetamines and cocaine
   c. Nicotine
   d. Opioids
   e. CNS depressants

IV. Organic Mental Disorders
   A. The DMS-III-R identifies the following categories of organic mental disorders:
      1. Dementias arising in the senium and presenium.
         a. Primary degenerative dementia of the Alzheimer type.
         b. Multi-infarct dementia
      2. Psychoactive substance-induced organic mental disorders.
      3. Organic mental disorders associated with physical disorders or conditions, or whose etiology is unknown.
   B. Dementias arising in the senium and presenium.
      1. Primary degenerative dementia of the Alzheimer type.
         a. Characterized by the syndrome of dementia.
         b. Onset is slow and insidious and the course of the disorder is generally progressive and deteriorating.
         c. Definitive diagnosis can only be made by brain biopsy or autopsy examination.
         d. Predisposing factors
            (1) Acetylcholine alterations
            (2) Accumulation of aluminum
            (3) Alterations in the immune system

                (4) Head trauma
                (5) Genetic factors
        2. Multi-infarct dementia
            a. Dementia due to significant cerebrovascular disease (significant number of small strokes).
            b. More abrupt onset than Alzheimer type, and course is more variable.
            c. Predisposing factors
                (1) Arterial hypertension
                (2) Cerebral emboli
                (3) Cerebral thrombosis
    C. Psychoactive substance-induced organic mental disorders
        1. These disorders are identified by various syndromes of symptoms caused by the direct effects of various psychoactive substances on the central nervous system. The classes of substances that most commonly induce these organic syndromes include:
            a. Alcohol
            b. Amphetamines and related substances
            c. Caffeine
            d. Cannabis
            e. Cocaine
            f. Hallucinogens
            g. Inhalants
            h. Nicotine
            i. Opioids
            j. Phencyclidine and related substances
            k. Sedatives, hypnotics, or anxiolytics
        2. Predisposing factors
            a. Prolonged heavy use of substances that are taken nonmedicinally to alter mood or behavior.
    D. Organic mental disorders associated with physical disorders or conditions, or whose etiology is unknown
        1. Dementia is the most common syndrome of symptoms associated with these disorders, although in severe acute infections, the clinical picture is more likely to be that of delirium.
        2. Predisposing factors
            a. Parkinson's Disease
            b. Huntington's Chorea
            c. Pick's Disease
            d. Multiple Sclerosis
            e. Epilepsy
            f. Neurosyphilis
            g. Head trauma
            h. Other medical conditions
            i. Frontal or temporal lobe lesions
            j. CNS or systemic infections
            k. Acquired Immunodeficiency Syndrome
V. Application of the Nursing Process
    A. Assessment is conducted through acquiring a patient history, physical assessment, and diagnostic laboratory evaluations.
    B. Nursing diagnoses are formulated from data gathered during the assessment.
    C. Nursing intervention is aimed at protection from injury, maintaining orientation, accomplishing activities of daily living, and providing support for caregivers outside the hospital.
VI. Medical Treatment Modalities
    A. Psychopharmacology
        1. In progressive degenerative dementia.
        2. In psychoactive substance-induced intoxication or withdrawal.
VII. Summary
VIII. Review Questions

126

LEARNING ACTIVITY

ORGANIC MENTAL DISORDERS

Circle whether each of the following organic mental disorders is acute or chronic (A or C) and reversible or irreversible (R or I).

1.	Primary Degenerative Dementia of the Alzheimer Type	A	C	R	I
2.	Multi-Infarct Dementia	A	C	R	I
3.	Alcohol-Induced Withdrawal	A	C	R	I
4.	Nicotine-Induced Withdrawal	A	C	R	I
5.	Alcohol-Induced Delirium	A	C	R	I
6.	Alcohol-Induced Dementia	A	C	R	I
7.	Dementia associated with uncontrolled epilepsy	A	C	R	I
8.	PCP-Induced Hallucinations	A	C	R	I
9.	Organic Mood Disorder related to amphetamine withdrawal	A	C	R	I
10.	Delirium associated with inhalant intoxication	A	C	R	I

ORGANIC MENTAL SYNDROMES

Delirium

Dementia

Amnestic Syndrome

Organic Hallucinosis

Organic Delusional Syndrome

Organic Mood Syndrome

Organic Anxiety Syndrome

Organic Personality Syndrome

Intoxication

Withdrawal

ORGANIC MENTAL DISORDERS:

DEMENTIAS ARISING IN THE SENIUM AND PRESENIUM

1. Primary degenerative dementia of the Alzheimer type.

2. Multi-infarct dementia

PSYCHOACTIVE SUBSTANCE-INDUCED ORGANIC MENTAL DISORDERS

Alcohol

Amphetamines and Related Substances

Caffeine

Cannabis

Cocaine

Hallucinogens

Inhalants

Nicotine

Opioids

Phencyclidine and Related Substances

Sedatives, Hypnotics or Anxiolytics

ORGANIC MENTAL DISORDERS ASSOCIATED WITH PHYSICAL DISORDERS OR CONDITIONS, OR WHOSE ETIOLOGY IS UNKNOWN

Parkinson's Disease

Huntington's Chorea

Pick's Disease

Multiple Sclerosis

Epilepsy

Neurosyphilis

Head Trauma

Frontal or Temporal Lobe Lesions

CNS or Systemic Infections

Acquired Immunodeficiency Syndrome

NURSING DIAGNOSIS FOR PATIENTS WITH ORGANIC MENTAL SYNDROMES AND DISORDERS

1. Potential for Injury related to CNS agitation from substance withdrawal.

2. Potential for Trauma related to impaired cognition and disorientation.

3. Altered Thought Processes related to cerebral degeneration.

4. Altered Nutrition: Less than body requirements related to poor diet or malabsorption from chronic substance abuse.

5. Self-care deficit related to disorientation, confusion, and memory deficits.

CHAPTER 17: PSYCHOACTIVE SUBSTANCE USE DISORDERS

CHAPTER FOCUS

The focus of this chapter is on individuals with psychoactive substance use disorders. Symptomatology and predisposing factors are discussed. Role of the nurse in the care of these patients is emphasized.

LEARNING OBJECTIVES

After reading this chapter, the student will be able to:

1. Differentiate between *abuse* and *dependence*.
2. Discuss predisposing factors implicated in the etiology of substance use disorders.
3. Identify symptomatology and use the information in assessment of patients with various substance use disorders.
4. Identify nursing diagnoses common to patients with substance use disorders and select appropriate nursing interventions for each.
5. Describe relevant criteria for evaluating nursing care of patients with substance use disorders.
6. Discuss the issue of substance abuse and dependence within the profession of nursing.
7. Define *co-dependency* and identify behavioral characteristics associated with the disorder.
8. Discuss treatment of co-dependency.
9. Describe various modalities relevant to treatment of individuals with substance use disorders.

KEY TERMS

abuse
dependence
Wernicke's encephalopathy
Korsakoff's psychosis
ascites
esophageal varices

hepatic encephalopathy
peer assistance programs
co-dependency
Alcoholics Anonymous
disulfiram

CHAPTER OUTLINE/LECTURE NOTES

I. Introduction
   A. Psychoactive substance use disorders refer to the maladaptive behavior associated with regular use of the substances.
   B. Some illegal substances have achieved a degree of social acceptance by various sub-cultural groups within our society.
II. Psychoactive Substance Dependence
   A. Physical dependence. Criteria for identifying physical dependence:
      1. Consumes more substance than intended.
      2. Unsuccessful attempts to reduce or control use.
      3. Spends a lot of time in efforts to procure the drug.
      4. Intoxication or withdrawal syndrome interferes with activities of daily living.
      5. Uses substance during physically hazardous activities.
      6. Uses substance rather than participate in usual activities.
      7. Uses substance despite knowledge that a problem exists or is exacerbated by its use.
      8. Significant tolerance develops.
      9. Characteristic withdrawal symptoms develop with cessation or reduction of the substance.
      10. The substance is often taken to relieve or avoid withdrawal symptoms.

B. Psychological dependence. Exists when an individual believes that use of a substance is necessary to maintain an optimal state of personal well-being, interpersonal relations, or skill performance.

III. Psychoactive Substance Abuse
   A. Criteria for identifying substance abuse:
      1. Continued use despite knowledge of having a persistent or recurrent social, occupational, psychological, or physical problem that is caused or exacerbated by use of the substance.
      2. Recurrent use in situations in which use is physically hazardous.

IV. Classes of Psychoactive Substances
   A. Alcohol
   B. Amphetamines and related substances
   C. Cannabis
   D. Cocaine
   E. Hallucinogens
   F. Inhalants
   G. Nicotine
   H. Opioids
   I. Phencyclidine and related substances
   J. Sedatives, hypnotics, or anxiolytics

V. Predisposing Factors
   A. Biological factors
      1. Genetics. Apparent hereditary factor, particularly with alcoholism.
      2. Biochemical. Alcohol may produce morphinelike substances in the brain that are responsible for alcohol addiction.
   B. Psychological factors
      1. Developmental influences. May relate to severe ego impairment and disturbances in the sense of self.
      2. Personality factors. Certain personality traits have been suggested to play a part in both the development and maintenance of alcohol dependence. They include: impulsivity, negative self-concept, weak ego, low social conformity, neuroticism, and introversion.
   C. Sociocultural factors
      1. Social learning. Children and adolescents are more likely to use substances if they have parents who provide a model for substance use. Use of substances may also be promoted within one's peer group.
      2. Conditioning. Pleasurable effects from substance use act as a positive reinforcement for their continued use.
      3. Cultural and ethnic influences. Some cultures are more prone to use of substances than others.

VI. The Dynamics of Psychoactive Substance Use Disorders
   A. Alcohol Abuse and Dependence
      1. A profile of the substance
      2. Historical aspects
      3. Patterns of use/abuse
         a. Phase I. The Prealcoholic Phase
         b. Phase II. The Early Alcoholic Phase
         c. Phase III. The Crucial Phase
         d. Phase IV. The Chronic Phase
      4. Effects on the Body
         a. Peripheral neuropathy
         b. Alcoholic myopathy
         c. Wernicke's encephalopathy
         d. Korsakoff's psychosis
         e. Alcoholic cardiomyopathy
         f. Esophagitis
         g. Gastritis
         h. Pancreatitis
         i. Alcoholic hepatitis
         j. Cirrhosis of the liver
            (1) portal hypertension
            (2) ascites
            (3) esophageal varices

134

(4) hepatic encephalopathy
- k. Leukopenia
- l. Thrombocytopenia
- m. Sexual dysfunction
- B. Other CNS depressant abuse and dependence
    1. A profile of the substance
        - a. Barbiturates
        - b. Non-barbiturate hypnotics
        - c. Antianxiety agents
    2. Historical aspects
    3. Patterns of use/abuse
    4. Effects on the body
        - a. Effects on sleep and dreaming
        - b. Respiratory depression
        - c. Cardiovascular effects
        - d. Renal function
        - e. Hepatic effects
        - f. Body temperature
        - g. Sexual functioning
- C. CNS stimulant abuse and dependence
    1. A profile of the substance
        - a. Amphetamines
        - b. Non-amphetamine stimulants
        - c. Cocaine
        - d. Caffeine
        - e. Nicotine
    2. Historical aspects
    3. Patterns of use/abuse
    4. Effects on the body
        - a. CNS effects
        - b. Cardiovascular/pulmonary effects
        - c. Gastrointestinal and renal effects
        - d. Sexual functioning
- D. Opioid abuse and dependence
    1. A profile of the substance
        - a. Opioids of natural origin
        - b. Opioid derivatives
        - c. Synthetic opiate-like drugs
    2. Historical aspects
    3. Patterns of use/abuse
    4. Effects on the body
        - a. Central nervous system
        - b. Gastrointestinal effects
        - c. Cardiovascular effects
        - d. Sexual functioning
- E. Hallucinogen abuse and dependence
    1. A profile of the substance
        - a. Naturally-occurring hallucinogens
            (1) mescaline
            (2) psilocybin and psilocyn
            (3) ololiuqui
        - b. Synthetic compounds
            (1) LSD
            (2) dimethyltryptamine
            (3) diethyltryptamine
            (4) STP
            (5) phencyclidine

(6) designer drugs
2. Historical aspects
3. Patterns of use/abuse
4. Effects on the body
F. Cannabis abuse and dependence
1. A profile of the substance
a. Marijuana
b. Hashish
2. Historical aspects
3. Patterns of use/abuse
4. Effects on the body
a. Cardiovascular effects
b. Respiratory effects
c. Reproductive effects
d. Central nervous system effects
e. Sexual functioning
VII. Application of the Nursing Function
A. Nurse must begin relationship development with a substance abuser by examining own attitudes and drinking habits.
B. Various assessment tools are available for determining the extent of a patient's problem with substances.
1. Michigan Alcoholism Screening Test (MAST)
2. CAGE Questionnaire
C. Nursing diagnoses are formulated from the data gathered during the assessment phase. Outcome criteria are established for each.
D. Nursing intervention for the patient with substance use disorder is aimed at acceptance of use of substances as a problem, acceptance of personal responsibility for use of substances, identification of more adaptive coping strategies, and restoration of nutritional status.
VIII. The Impaired Nurse
A. It is estimated that there are about 40,000 alcoholic nurses in the U.S., and that narcotic addiction among nurses is 30 to 100 times greater than it is in the general population.
B. Clues that may identify an impaired nurse:
1. May appear happy or sad.
2. May have increased appetite or no appetite at all.
3. May be verbal and energetic, or slow thinking with impaired concentration.
4. May volunteer to work extra shifts.
5. May leave the floor a lot or spend a great deal of time in the restroom.
6. May be more accidents or unusual occurrences reported when impaired nurse is on duty.
7. More patients may complain of pain and insomnia even though many narcotic analgesics and sedatives are documented as administered.
8. As the impairment progresses, there may be inaccurate drug counts, increased vial breakage and drug wastage, and discrepancies in documentation.
9. Lapses in memory may occur.
10. Personal appearance and job performance will likely be affected.
C. Peer Assistance Program developed by the American Nurses' Association in 1982.
1. To assist impaired nurses to recognize their impairment.
2. To obtain necessary treatment.
3. To regain accountability within their profession.
4. Contract is drawn up:
a. To detail method of treatment.
b. To establish guidelines for monitoring course of treatment.
5. Usually lasts for a period of two years.
IX. Co-Dependency
A. Defined as an exaggerated dependent pattern of learned behaviors, beliefs, and feelings that make life painful. It is dependence on people and things outside the self, along with neglect of the self to the point of having little self-identity.
B. Derives self-worth from others.
C. Feels responsible for the happiness of others.

D. Denial that problems exist is common.

E. Feelings are kept in control, and anxiety may be released in the form of stress-related illnesses, or compulsive behaviors such as eating, spending, working, or use of substances.

F. The Co-Dependent Nurse

    1. Certain characteristics associated with co-dependency seem to apply to some nurses who often have a tendency to fulfill everyone's needs but their own.

        a. Caretaking. Meeting the needs of others to the point of neglecting their own.

        b. Perfectionism. Low self-esteem and fear of failure drives co-dependent nurses to strive for an unrealistic level of achievement.

        c. Denial. A refusal to acknowledge that any personal problems or painful issues exist.

        d. Poor communication. Co-dependent nurses rarely express their true feelings.

G. Treating co-dependence

    1. Stage I. The Survival Stage. Letting go of the denial that problems exist.

    2. Stage II. The Re-identification Stage. Taking responsibility for own dysfunctional behavior.

    3. Stage III. The Core Issues Stage. Facing the fact that relationships cannot be managed by force or will.

    4. Stage IV. The Re-integration Stage. Accepting self and willingness to change.

X. Treatment Modalities for Substance Use Disorders

A. Alcoholics Anonymous

B. Various support groups patterned after Alcoholics Anonymous, but for individuals with problems with other substances.

C. Alcohol deterrent therapy

D. Counseling

E. Group therapy

XI. Summary

XII. Review Questions

LEARNING ACTIVITY

SYMPTOMS ASSOCIATED WITH PSYCHOACTIVE SUBSTANCES

Fill in the spaces provided with the most common examples and symptoms of substance abuse disorders of which the nurse should be aware.

Drugs	Symptoms of Use	Symptoms of Intoxication	Symptoms of Withdrawal
CNS depressants Examples:			
CNS stimulants Examples:			
Opioids Examples:			
Hallucinogens Examples:			
Cannabis Examples:			

CLASSES OF PSYCHOACTIVE SUBSTANCES

Alcohol

Amphetamines and Related Substances

Cannabis

Cocaine

Hallucinogens

Inhalants

Nicotine

Opioids

Phencyclidine and Related Substances

**Sedatives, Hypnotics, or
Anxiolytics**

PREDISPOSING FACTORS TO SUBSTANCE USE DISORDER

BIOLOGICAL FACTORS

Genetics
Biochemical

PSYCHOLOGICAL FACTORS

Developmental Influences
Personality Factors

SOCIOCULTURAL FACTORS

Social Learning
Conditioning
Cultural and Ethnic Influences

NURSING DIAGNOSES COMMON
TO PATIENTS WITH
SUBSTANCE USE DISORDERS

1. Ineffective denial related to weak, underdeveloped ego.

2. Ineffective individual coping related to inadequate coping skills and weak ego.

3. Altered nutrition: less than body requirements related to poor diet (takes substances rather than eating).

4. Potential for infection related to malnutrition and altered immune condition.

5. Self-esteem disturbance related to weak ego and lack of positive feedback.

6. Knowledge deficit (effects of substance abuse on the body) related to denial of problems with substances.

CO-DEPENDENT BEHAVIORS

1. Fulfills others' needs while neglecting own.

2. Anxiety and boundary distortions around intimacy and separation.

3. Enmeshment in relationships with personality disordered, chemically dependent, or impulse disordered individuals.

4. Denial of problems and constriction of emotions.

5. Depression, anxiety, substance abuse.

6. Stress-related medical illnesses.

KEY WORDS
AND CONCEPTS

Abuse

Physical Dependence

Psychological Dependence

Tolerance

Intoxication

Withdrawal

Impaired Nurse

Co-dependency

Deterrent Therapy

CHAPTER 18:   SCHIZOPHRENIC, DELUSIONAL, AND RELATED PSYCHOTIC DISORDERS

CHAPTER FOCUS

The focus of this chapter is on nursing care of the patient with psychotic disorders.   Predisposing factors and symptomatology are explored, and nursing care is presented in the context of the five steps of the nursing process. Medical treatment modalities are also discussed.

LEARNING OBJECTIVES

After reading this chapter, the student will be able to:

1.   Discuss the concept of schizophrenic, delusional, and related psychotic disorders.
2.   Identify predisposing factors in the development of these disorders.
3.   Describe various types of schizophrenic, delusional, and related psychotic disorders.
4.   Identify symptomatology associated with these disorders and use this information in patient assessment.
5.   Describe appropriate nursing interventions for behaviors associated with these disorders.
6.   Describe relevant criteria for evaluating nursing care of patients with schizophrenic, delusional, and related psychotic disorders.
7.   Discuss various modalities relevant to treatment of schizophrenic, delusional, and related psychotic disorders.

KEY TERMS

delusions	hallucinations
double-bind communication	catatonia
paranoia	religiosity
magical thinking	associative looseness
meologism	clang association
word salad	circumstantiality
tangentiality	perseveration
illusion	echolalia
echopraxia	autism
waxy flexibility	anhedonia
social skills training	neuroleptic

CHAPTER OUTLINE/LECTURE NOTES

I.   Introduction
   A. The word schizophrenia is derived from the Greek words "skhizo" (split) and "phren" (mind).
   B. Schizophrenia is probably caused by a combination of factors, including genetic predisposition, biochemical dysfunction, and psychosocial stress.
   C. Schizophrenia requires treatment that is comprehensive and is presented in a multidisciplinary effort.
   D. Schizophrenia probably causes more lengthy hospitalizations, more chaos in family life, more exorbitant costs to individuals and governments, and more fears than any other mental illness.
II.   Nature of the Disorder
   A. Schizophrenia results in disturbances in thought processes, perception, and affect.
   B. There is severe deterioration of social and occupational functioning.
   C. Approximately 1% of the population will develop schizophrenia over the course of a lifetime.
   D. The premorbid behavior of an individual with schizophrenia can be viewed in four phases.

1. Phase I - The Schizoid Personality. Indifferent, cold, and aloof, these individuals are loners. They do not enjoy close relationships with others.
2. Phase II - The Prodromal Phase. In this phase, the individuals are socially withdrawn and have behavior that is peculiar or eccentric. Role functioning is impaired, personal hygiene is neglected, and disturbances exist in communication, ideation, and perception.
3. Phase III - Schizophrenia. In the active phase of the disorder, psychotic symptoms are prominent. These include delusions, hallucinations, and impairment in work, social relations, and self-care.
4. Phase IV - Residual Phase. Symptoms similar to the prodromal phase, with flat affect and impairment in role functioning being prominent.

III. Predisposing Factors
   A. Genetic influences. A growing body of knowledge indicates that genetics plays an important role in the development of schizophrenia.
   B. Biochemical influences. One theory suggests that schizophrenia may be caused by an excess of dopamine-dependent neuronal activity in the brain. Abnormalities in the neurotransmitters norepinephrine, serotonin, acetylcholine, and gamma-aminobutyric acid have also been suggested.
   C. Physiological influences. Several physiological factors have been implicated, including viral infection, brain abnormalities, and histological changes in the brain. Various physical conditions, such as epilepsy, systemic lupus erythematosus, myxedema, Parkinsonism, and Wilson's disease, have also been implicated.
   D. Psychological influences. Poor early relationship between mother and child has been suggested as a predisposing factor by several psychodynamic theorists. Dysfunctional family system and double-bind communication have also been suggested.
   E. Environmental influences. Lower socioeconomic status has been linked to the development of schizophrenia. Stressful life events have been associated with the onset of schizophrenic symptoms. Responses vary according to the number and severity of life events and the degree of vulnerability to the impact of the life event.
   F. The transactional model. Schizophrenia is likely the result of a combination of biological, psychological, and environmental influences on an individual who is vulnerable to the illness.

IV. Types of Schizophrenic and Other Psychotic Disorders
   A. Disorganized schizophrenia. Chronic variety with flat or inappropriate affect. Silliness and incongruous giggling is common. Behavior is bizarre, and social interaction is impaired.
   B. Catatonic schizophrenia.
      1. Catatonic stupor. Characterized by extreme psychomotor retardation. Patient is usually mute. Posturing is common.
      2. Catatonic excitement. Extreme psychomotor agitation. Purposeless movements that must be curtailed to prevent injury to patient or others.
   C. Paranoid schizophrenia. Characterized by paranoid delusions. Patient may be argumentative, hostile, and aggressive.
   D. Undifferentiated schizophrenia. Bizarre behavior that does not meet the criteria outlined for the other types of schizophrenia. Delusions and hallucinations are prominent.
   E. Residual schizophrenia. This category is used with the individual who has a history of at least one episode of schizophrenia with prominent psychotic symptoms. Also known as ambulatory schizophrenia, this is the stage that follows an acute disorder.
   F. Schizoaffective disorder. Schizophrenic symptoms accompanied by a strong element of symptomatology associated with the mood disorders, either mania or depression.
   G. Brief reactive psychosis. Sudden onset of psychotic symptoms following a severe psychosocial stressor. Symptoms last no more than one month, and the individual returns to the full premorbid level of functioning.
   H. Schizophreniform disorder. Same symptoms as schizophrenia with the exception that the duration of the disorder has been less than 6 months.
   I. Delusional disorder. The existence of prominent, nonbizarre delusions.
      1. Erotomanic type. The individual believes that someone, usually of a higher status, is in love with him or her.
      2. Grandiose type. Irrational ideas regarding own worth, talent, knowledge, or power.
      3. Jealous type. Irrational idea that the person's sexual partner is unfaithful.
      4. Persecutory type. The individual believes he or she is being malevolently treated in some way.
      5. Somatic type. The individual has an irrational belief that he or she has some physical defect, disorder, or disease.
   J. Induced psychotic disorder. A delusional system develops in a second person as a result of a close relationship

with another person who already has a psychotic disorder with prominent delusions.

V. Application of the Nursing Process
A. Background assessment data
   1. Content of thought
      a. Delusions - false personal beliefs.
      b. Religiosity - excessive demonstration of obsession with religious ideas and behavior.
      c. Paranoia - extreme suspiciousness of others.
      d. Magical thinking - the idea that if one thinks something it will be true.
   2. Form of thought
      a. Associative looseness - shift of ideas from one topic to another.
      b. Neologisms - made-up words that have meaning only to the individual who invents them.
      c. Concrete thinking - literal interpretations of the environment.
      d. Clang associations - choice of words is governed by sound (often rhyming).
      e. Word salad - a groups of words put together in a random fashion.
      f. Circumstantiality - a delay in reaching the point of a communication due to unnecessary and tedious details.
      g. Tangentiality - unable to get to point of communication due to introduction of many new topics.
      h. Mutism - inability or refusal to speak.
      i. Perseveration - persistent repetition of the same word or idea in response to different questions.
   3. Perception - the interpretation of stimuli through the senses.
      a. Hallucinations - false sensory perceptions not associated with real external stimuli.
      b. Illusions - misperceptions of real external stimuli.
   4. Affect - emotional tone
      a. Inappropriate affect - emotions are incongruent with the circumstances.
      b. Bland or flat - weak emotional tone.
      c. Apathy - disinterest in the environment.
   5. Sense of self - the uniqueness and individuality a person feels.
      a. Echolalia - repeating words that are heard.
      b. Echopraxia - repeating movements that are observed.
      c. Identification and imitation - taking on the form of behavior one observes in another.
      d. Depersonalization - feelings of unreality.
   6. Volition - impairment in the ability to initiate goal-directed activity.
      a. Emotional ambivalence - the coexistence of opposite emotions toward the same object.
   7. Impaired interpersonal functioning and relationship to the external world.
      a. Autism - focusing inward on a fantasy world, while distorting or excluding the external environment.
      b. Deteriorated appearance - personal grooming and self-care activities are impaired.
   8. Psychomotor behavior.
      a. Anergia - a deficiency of energy.
      b. Waxy flexibility - passive yielding of all moveable parts of the body to any efforts made at placing them in certain positions.
      c. Posturing - voluntary assumption of inappropriate or bizarre postures.
      d. Pacing and rocking - pacing back and forth and rocking of the body.
   9. Associated features
      a. Anhedonia - inability to experience pleasure.
      b. Regression - retreat to an earlier level of development.
B. Nursing diagnosis
   1. Alteration in thought processes
   2. Sensory-perceptual alteration: auditory/visual
   3. Social isolation
   4. Potential for violence: self or others
   5. Impaired verbal communication
   6. Self-care deficit
   7. Ineffective family coping: disabling
   8. Impaired home maintenance management
C. Planning/implementation
   1. Care plan for the patient with schizophrenia
   2. Outcome criteria

      2. Outcome criteria
   D. Evaluation
      1. Reassessment data on which to base the effectiveness of nursing actions.
VI.   Treatment Modalities for Schizophrenic and Other Psychotic Disorders
   A. Psychological treatments
      1. Individual psychotherapy - long-term therapeutic approach; difficult because of patient's impairment in interpersonal functioning.
      2. Group therapy - some success if occurring over the long-term course of the illness; less successful in acute treatment.
      3. Behavior therapy - chief drawback has been the inability to generalize to the community setting once the patient has been discharged from the hospital.
      4. Social skills training - the use of role play to teach patient appropriate eye contact, interpersonal skills, voice intonation, posture, etc., aimed at improvement in relationship development.
   B. Social treatment
      1. Milieu therapy - best if used in conjunction with psychopharmacology.
      2. Family therapy - aimed at helping family members cope with the long-term effects of the illness.
   C. Organic treatment
      1. Psychopharmacology
         a. Antipsychotics - used to decrease agitation and psychotic symptoms.
         b. Antiparkinsonian agents - used to counteract the extrapyramidal symptoms associated with antipsychotic medications.
         c. Others - reserpine, lithium carbonate, carbamazepine, valium, and propranolol have been used with mixed results.
VII.   Summary
VIII. Review Questions

LEARNING ACTIVITIES

Match the behaviors on the right to the appropriate terminology listed on the left.

_____ 1. autism

_____ 2. mutism

_____ 3. hallucination

_____ 4. persecutory delusion

_____ 5. word salad

_____ 6. religiosity

_____ 7. associative looseness

_____ 8. inappropriate affect

_____ 9. paranoia

_____ 10. magical thinking

_____ 11. neologism

_____ 12. clang association

_____ 13. waxy flexibility

_____ 14. regression

_____ 15. delusion of grandeur

a. Kneels to pray in front of water fountain; prays during group therapy and during other group activities.

b. Refuses to eat food that comes on tray, stating, "They are trying to poison me."

c. "When I get out of the hospital I'm going to buy me a sprongle."

d. Does not talk.

e. Keeps arm in position nurse left it after taking blood pressure. Assumed this position for hours.

f. "When I speak, presidents and kings listen."

g. A withdrawal inward into one's own fantasy world.

h. "I'm going to the circus. Jesus is God. The police are playing for keeps."

i. "We can't close the drapes, for if we do, the sun won't shine."

j. "Test, test, this is a test. I do not jest; we get no rest."

k. Laughs when told that his or her mother has just died.

l. In response to stressful situation, begins to suck thumb and soils clothing.

m. "Get by for anyone just to answer fortune cookies."

n. "If the FBI finds me here, I'll never get out alive."

o. Stops talking in mid-sentence, tilts head to side, and listens.

CASE STUDY

Read the following case study and fill in the blanks with the description of the information that is underlined and numbered in the text.

Sandra was a 37-year-old woman who was picked up by the police after she ran away from her parents' home. Sandra has a history of paranoid schizophrenia for 17 years. She has had numerous hospitalizations.

Police were called when Sandra began wandering through a local park and screaming at everyone, "I know you are possessed by the devil!" During her initial interview, she is very guarded and suspicious of the nurse (1). "I can read your mind, you know" (2).

Sandra is assigned to a room and oriented to the unit. At 5:00 p.m., the nurse says to Sandra, "Sandra, it's time for dinner." Sandra responds, "Time for dinner; time for dinner; time for dinner" (3). The nurse notices that each time she wipes her mouth with her napkin at dinner, Sandra does the same (4).

Sandra's mother reports that Sandra stopped taking her medicine about a month ago, stating, "When you don't have a brain (5), you don't need brain medicine." Shortly afterward, she became totally despondent, taking no pleasure in activities she had always found enjoyable (6). She stayed in her room, sitting on her bed moving back and forth in a slow, rhythmic fashion (7). Sometimes she would not even get up to go to the bathroom, instead soiling herself in an infantile manner (8). She seemed to experience a total lack of energy for usual activities of daily living (9).

On the unit, Sandra appears disinterested in everything around her (10). She sits alone, talking and laughing to herself (11). At one point, she hears a laugh track on TV and states, "They're laughing at me. I know they are" (12).

Sandra's anxiety level starts to rise. She begins to pace the floor. Her agitation increases and she finally picks up a chair and hurls it toward the nurses' station, yelling, "The devil says all blonds must be annihilated!"

What would be Sandra's priority nursing diagnosis?

What medication would you expect the physician to order for Sandra?

For what adverse effects would you be on the alert with this drug?

In what developmental stage (Erikson) would you place Sandra? Why?

Theoretically, in what developmental stage *should* she be?

(1) ___paranoia___

(2) _____

(3) _____

(4) _____

(5) _____

(6) _____

(7) _____

(8) _____

(9) _____

(10) _____

(11) _____

(12) _____

149

CLINICAL EXERCISE

In lieu of a care plan, have students construct a Critical Pathway of Care for a patient with schizophrenia. Instead of the standard CPC, have the student write time dimensions to fit the days he or she will be on the clinical unit. Goals should be of the type that may be achieved during the clinical rotation time.

PREDISPOSING FACTORS TO SCHIZOPHRENIA

GENETIC INFLUENCES
Twin Studies
Adoption Studies

BIOCHEMICAL INFLUENCES
Dopamine Hypothesis
Others

PHYSIOLOGIC INFLUENCES
Viral Infection
Anatomical Abnormalities
Histological Changes
Physical Conditions

PSYCHOLOGIC INFLUENCES
Mother-Child Relationship
Dysfunctional Family System
Double-Bind Communication

ENVIRONMENTAL INFLUENCES
Socio-Cultural Factors
Stressful Life Events

THE TRANSACTIONAL MODEL

TYPES OF SCHIZOPHRENIA AND OTHER PSYCHOTIC DISORDERS

Disorganized Schizophrenia

Catatonic Schizophrenia

Paranoid Schizophrenia

Undifferentiated Schizophrenia

Residual Schizophrenia

Schizoaffective Disorder

Brief Reactive Psychosis

Schizophreniform Disorder

Delusional Disorder

Induced Psychotic Disorder

SYMPTOMS OF SCHIZOPHRENIA

CONTENT OF THOUGHT
Delusions
Religiosity
Paranoia
Magical Thinking

FORM OF THOUGHT
Neologisms
Concrete Thinking
Clang Associations
Word Salad
Circumstantiality
Tangentiality
Mutism
Perserveration

PERCEPTION
Hallucinations
Illusions

AFFECT
Inappropriate Affect
Bland or Flat Affect
Apathy

SENSE OF SELF
Echolalia
Echopraxia
Identification/Imitation
Depersonalization

VOLITION
Emotional Ambivalence

IMPAIRED INTERPERSONAL FUNCTIONING AND RELATIONSHIP TO THE EXTERNAL WORLD
Autism
Deteriorated Appearance

PSYCHOMOTOR BEHAVIOR
Anergia
Waxy Flexibility
Posturing
Pacing and Rocking

ASSOCIATED FEATURES
Anhedonia
Regression

NURSING DIAGNOSES
FOR
SCHIZOPHRENIA

Altered Thought Processes

**Sensory-Perceptual Alteration:
Auditory/Visual**

Social Isolation

**Potential for Violence:
Self or Others**

Impaired Verbal Communication

Self-Care Deficit

**Ineffective Family Coping:
Disabling**

Altered Health Maintenance

**Impaired Home Maintenance
Management**

CHAPTER 19: MOOD DISORDERS

CHAPTER FOCUS

The focus of this chapter is on nursing care of the patient with mood disorders (depression or mania). Predisposing factors and symptomatology are explored, and nursing care is presented in the context of the five steps of the nursing process. Medical treatment modalities are also discussed.

LEARNING OBJECTIVES

After reading this chapter, the student will be able to:

1. Recount historical perspectives of mood disorders.
2. Discuss epidemiological statistics related to mood disorders.
3. Differentiate between normal and maladaptive responses to loss.
4. Describe various types of mood disorders.
5. Identify predisposing factors in the development of mood disorders.
6. Discuss implications of depression related to developmental stage.
7. Identify symptomatology associated with mood disorders and use this information in patient assessment.
8. Formulate nursing diagnoses and goals of care for patients with mood disorders.
9. Describe appropriate nursing interventions for behaviors associated with mood disorders.
10. Describe relevant criteria for evaluating nursing care of patients with mood disorders.
11. Discuss various modalities relevant to treatment of mood disorders.
12. Discuss incidence, prevalence, and risk factors related to suicide.
13. Describe predisposing factors implicated in the etiology of suicide.
14. Differentiate between facts and fables regarding suicide.
15. Apply the nursing process to individuals exhibiting suicidal behavior.

KEY TERMS

anticipatory grieving
altruistic suicide
anomic suicide
bereavement overload
bipolar disorder
cognitive therapy
cyclothymia
delayed grief
delirious mania
dysthymia
egoistic suicide

exaggerated grief
grief
hypomania
mania
melancholia
mood
mourning
postpartum depression
prolonged grief
psychomotor retardation
tyramine

CHAPTER OUTLINE/LECTURE NOTES

I.   Introduction
     A. Depression is the oldest and most frequently described psychiatric illness.
     B. Transient symptoms are normal, healthy responses to everyday disappointments in life.
     C. Pathological depression occurs when adaptation is ineffective.
     D. Suicide as a coping strategy closely associated with mood disorders is discussed.
     E. Various medical treatment modalities are explored.

II. Historical Perspectives
    A. Many ancient cultures have believed in the supernatural or divine origin of depression and mania.
    B. Hippocrates believed that melancholia was caused by an excess of black bile, a heavily toxic substance produced in the spleen or intestine, which affected the brain.
    C. Various other theories were espoused regarding the etiology of depression. It was described as the result of obstruction of vital air circulation, excessive brooding, or helpless situations beyond the patient's control.
    D. Nineteenth century definitions of mania narrowed it down to a disorder of affect and action.
    E. The perspectives of twentieth century theorists lend support to the notion of multiple causation in the development of mood disorders.
III. Epidemiology
    A. Ten to fourteen million Americans are afflicted with some form of major affective disorder.
    B. The worldwide annual prevalence rate for depression is 3 to 5%--approximately 100 million people.
    C. Gender. Depression is more prevalent in women than men. Bipolar disorder is roughly equal.
    D. Age. Depression is more common in young women and has a tendency to decrease with age. The opposite is true with men. Studies regarding bipolar disorder are inconsistent.
    E. Social class. There is an inverse relationship between social class and report of depressive symptoms. The opposite is true with bipolar disorder.
    F. Race. No consistent relationship between race and affective disorder has been reported.
    G. Marital status. Single and divorced persons are more likely to experience depression than married persons.
    H. Seasonality. Affective disorders are more prevalent in the spring and in the fall.
IV. The Grief Response
    A. Loss is an experience in which an individual relinquishes a connection to a valued object (animate/inanimate; a relationship or situation; or even a change or failure [real or perceived]).
    B. Stages of grief
        1. Elizabeth Kubler-Ross
            a. Denial
            b. Anger
            c. Bargaining
            d. Depression
            e. Acceptance
        2. John Bowlby
            a. Numbness/protest
            b. Disequilibrium
            c. Disorganization and despair
            d. Reorganization
        3. George Engel
            a. Shock and disbelief
            b. Developing awareness
            c. Restitution
            d. Resolution of the loss
            e. Recovery
    C. Length of the grief process
        1. Resolution is thought to have occurred when a bereaved individual is able to remember comfortably and realistically both pleasures and disappointments associated with that which has been lost.
        2. Several factors influence length of the grief process.
            a. Importance of the lost object as a source of support.
            b. Degree of dependency on the relationship with the lost object.
            c. Degree of ambivalence felt toward the lost object.
            d. Number and nature of other meaningful relationships the mourner has.
            e. Number and nature of previous grief experiences.
            f. Age of a lost person is influential.
            g. Health of the mourner at the time of loss.
            h. Degree of preparation for the loss.
    D. Anticipatory Grief
        1. The initiation and process of grieving before the significant loss actually occurs.
        2. Thought to facilitate the actual grief response when the loss occurs.
V. Maladaptive Responses to Loss

A. Types
   1. Delayed or inhibited grief. The absence of evidence of grief when it ordinarily would be expected.
      a. Can be considered pathological because the person does not deal with the reality of the loss.
   2. Prolonged grief. Exists when there has been no resumption of normal activities of daily living within four to eight weeks of a loss.
   3. Exaggerated grief response. A distorted grief reaction in which all of the symptoms associated with normal grieving are exaggerated out of proportion.
      a. Depressive mood disorder is a type of distorted grief reaction.
B. Normal vs. maladaptive grieving
   1. One crucial difference between normal and maladaptive grieving: the loss of self-esteem.
   2. The loss of self-esteem that almost invariably occurs in depression is not present with normal grief.
VI. Types of Mood Disorders
   A. Depressive disorders
      1. Major depression, single episode or recurrent
         a. With psychotic features
         b. Melancholic type
         c. Chronic
         d. Seasonal pattern
      2. Dysthymia
         a. Primary or secondary type
         b. Early or late onset
   B. Bipolar disorders
      1. Bipolar disorder, mixed
      2. Bipolar disorder, depressed
      3. Bipolar disorder, manic
      4. Cyclothymia
VII. Depressive Disorders
   A. Predisposing factors
      1. Biologic theories
         a. Genetics. Hereditary factor may be involved.
         b. Biochemical influences. Deficiency or norepinephrine, serotonin, and dopamine have been implicated.
         c. Neuroendocrine disturbances
            (1) Possible failure within the hypothalamic-pituitary-adrenocortical axis.
            (2) Possible diminished release of thyroid-stimulating hormone.
         d. Physiologic influences
            (1) Medication side-effects
            (2) Neurological disorders
            (3) Electrolyte disturbances
            (4) Hormonal disorders
            (5) Nutritional deficiencies
      2. Psychosocial theories
         a. Psychoanalytic theories
            (1) Freud: a loss is internalized and becomes directed against the ego.
            (2) Klein: the result of a poor mother-infant relationship.
         b. Learning theory
            (1) Learned helplessness: the individual who experiences numerous failures learns to give up trying.
         c. Object loss theory
            (1) Occurs when an individual is separated from a significant other during the first six months of life.
         d. Cognitive theory
            (1) Theory that cognitive distortions result in negative, defeatist attitudes that serve as the basis for depression.
         e. Transactional model. Exact etiology of depression remains unclear. Evidence continues to mount in support of multiple causation.
   B. Developmental implications
      1. Childhood depression
      2. Adolescent depression
      3. Senescence

4. Postpartum depression
C. Application of the nursing process to depressive disorders
   1. Background assessment data
      a. Symptoms occur by degree of severity and may be ranked as transient, mild, moderate, or severe.
      b. Transient: life's everyday disappointments that result in the "blues."
      c. Mild depression: identified with those symptoms of normal grieving.
      d. Moderate depression: identified by those symptoms associated with dysthymic disorder.
      e. Severe depression: identified by those symptoms associated with major depression and bipolar disorder, depressed.
   2. Nursing diagnoses are formulated by analyzing the data gathered during the assessment phase of the nursing process.
   3. Nursing interventions for the depressed patient are aimed at:
      a. Protection from harming self.
      b. Assisting with progression through the grief process.
      c. Enhancing patient self-esteem.
      d. Helping the patient determine ways to take control over his or her life.
      e. Assistance in confronting anger that has been turned inward on the self.
      f. Ensuring that needs related to nutrition, elimination, activity, rest, and personal hygiene are met.
   4. Outcome criteria are established for evaluating the effectiveness of nursing interventions.
VIII. Bipolar Disorder, Manic
   A. Predisposing factors
      1. Biologic theories
         a. Genetics. Strong hereditary implications.
         b. Biochemical influences. Possible excess of norepinephrine and dopamine.
         c. Electrolytes. Increased intracellular sodium and calcium has been implicated.
         d. Physiologic influences
            (1) Brain lesions
            (2) Medication side effects
      2. Psychosocial theories
         a. Psychoanalytic theories. Mania is viewed as a denial of, or defense against, depression.
         b. Theory of family dynamics. Views mania as the result of conditional love.
         c. The transactional model. Most likely occurs as the result of multiple influences.
   B. Application of the nursing process to bipolar disorder, manic.
      1. Background assessment data
         a. Symptoms may be categorized by degree of severity.
         b. Stage I. Hypomania. Symptoms not sufficiently severe to cause marked impairment in social or occupational functioning or to require hospitalization.
         c. Stage II. Acute Mania. Marked impairment in functioning of mood, cognition and perception, and activity and behavior. Usually requires hospitalization.
         d. Stage III. Delirious Mania. A grave form of the disorder characterized by severe clouding of consciousness and representing an intensification of the symptoms associated with acute mania.
      2. Nursing diagnoses are formulated by analyzing the data gathered during the assessment phase of the nursing process.
      3. Nursing interventions for the manic patient are aimed at:
         a. Protection from injury due to hyperactivity.
         b. Protection from harm for self and others.
         c. Restoration of nutritional status.
         d. Progression toward resolution of the grief process.
         e. Improvement in interactions with others.
         f. Acquiring sufficient rest and sleep.
      4. Outcome criteria are established for evaluating the effectiveness of nursing interventions.
IX. Treatment Modalities for Mood Disorders
   A. Psychological treatments
      1. Individual psychotherapy
      2. Group therapy
      3. Family therapy
      4. Cognitive therapy

B. Organic treatments
    1. Psychopharmacology
    2. Electroconvulsive therapy
X. Suicide
  A. Epidemiological factors
    1. Approximately 25,000 persons in the U.S. end their lives each year by suicide.
    2. Gender. Women attempt suicide more, but more men succeed.
    3. Age. Suicide risk and age are positively correlated.
    4. Religion. Protestants have significantly higher rates of suicide than Catholics or Jews.
    5. Socioeconomic status. Individuals in the very highest and lowest social classes have higher suicide rates than those in the middle classes.
    6. Race. Whites have suicide rates higher than those of Blacks.
    7. Other risk factors include mood disorders, severe insomnia, and family history of suicide.
XI. Predisposing Factors: Theories of Suicide
  A. Psychoanalytic theory. Suicide is viewed as a response to the intense self-hatred an individual possesses.
  B. Sociologic theory. Whether or not an individual commits suicide is determined by the degree of integration the individual feels within his or her society.
XII. Application of the Nursing Process with the Suicidal Patient
  A. An assessment is made emphasizing degree of risk, intent, plan, and availability of means.
  B. Nursing intervention is aimed at:
    1. Establishing a therapeutic relationship.
    2. Communicating the potential for suicide to team members.
    3. Staying with the person.
    4. Accepting the person.
    5. Listening to the person.
    6. Securing a no-suicide contract.
    7. Giving the person a message of hope.
    8. Giving the person something to do.
  C. Evaluation is based on achievement of outcome criteria.
XIII. Summary
XIV. Review Questions

LEARNING ACTIVITIES

SYMPTOMS OF MOOD DISORDERS

Beside each of the behaviors listed below, write the letter that identifies the disorder in which the behavior is most prevalent. The first one is completed as an example.

a. Dysthymia
b. Major depression
c. Transient depression

d. Cyclothymia
e. Bipolar disorder, manic
f. Delirious mania

___c___ 1. Feeling of the "blues" in response to everyday disappointments.

_____ 2. A clouding of consciousness occurs.

_____ 3. Outlook is gloomy and pessimistic.

_____ 4. Characterized by mood swings from hypomania to dysthymia.

_____ 5. Feelings of total despair and hopelessness.

_____ 6. Physical movement may come to a standstill.

_____ 7. Paranoid and grandiose delusions are common.

_____ 8. Feels at their best early in the morning and continually feels worse as the day progresses.

_____ 9. Excessive interest in sexual activity.

_____ 10. Carries out thoughts of self-destructive behavior.

_____ 11. Feels at their worst early in the morning and somewhat better as the day progresses.

_____ 12. Accelerated, pressured speech.

_____ 13. Frenzied motor activity characterized by agitated, purposeless movements.

FACTS AND FABLES ABOUT SUICIDE

Indicate with a T or F whether each of the following statements is true or false.

_____   1. Suicide is an inherited trait.

_____   2. Gunshot wounds are the leading cause of death among suicide victims.

_____   3. Most people give clues and warnings about their suicidal intentions.

_____   4. If a person has attempted suicide, he or she will not do it again.

_____   5. Suicide is the act of a psychotic person.

_____   6. Once a person is suicidal, he or she is suicidal forever.

_____   7. Most suicides occur when the severe depression has started to improve.

_____   8. Most suicidal people have ambivalent feelings about living and dying.

_____   9. If a suicidal person is intent upon dying, he or she cannot be stopped.

_____   10. People who talk about suicide don't commit suicide.

TYPES OF MOOD DISORDERS

MAJOR DEPRESSION
With Psychotic Features
Melancholic Type
Chronic
Seasonal Pattern

DYSTHYMIA
Secondary Type
Primary Type
Early or Late Onset

BIPOLAR DISORDER
Mixed
Manic
Depressed

CYCLOTHYMIA

SYMPTOMS OF DYSTHYMIA

Sadness, Dejection

Helplessness, Hopelessness

Flat Affect

Difficulty Experiencing Pleasure

Psychomotor Retardation

Slow Speech and Thinking

Self-Destructive Behavior

Anorexia or Overeating

Insomnia or Hypersomnia

Decreased Libido

Feels Best Early In The Morning

SYMPTOMS OF
MAJOR DEPRESSION

Total Despair

Hopelessness and Worthlessness

Absence of Emotional Tone

Inability to Experience Pleasure

Severe Psychomotor Retardation

Social Isolation

Delusions and Hallucinations

Lack of Energy to Carry Out Suicidal Ideas

General Slowdown of Body Processes

Feels Worst in the Morning

SYMPTOMS OF BIPOLAR, MANIC

Euphoria and Elation

Mood is Labile

Flight of Ideas

Loquaciousness

Paranoid and Grandiose Delusions

Excessive Psychomotor Activity

Sexually Uninhibited

Inexhaustible Energy

Diminished Sleep

Disorganized, Flamboyant, or
Bizarre Dress

CHAPTER 20: ANXIETY DISORDERS

CHAPTER FOCUS

The focus of this chapter is on nursing care of the patient with anxiety disorders. predisposing factors and symptomatology are explored, and nursing care is presented in the context of the five steps of the nursing process. Medical treatment modalities are also discussed.

LEARNING OBJECTIVES

After reading this chapter, the student will be able to:

1. Differentiate between the terms "stress," "anxiety," and "fear."
2. Discuss historical aspects and epidemiological statistics related to anxiety disorders.
3. Differentiate between "normal" anxiety and "psychoneurotic" anxiety.
4. Describe various types of anxiety disorders and identify symptomatology associated with each. Utilize this information in patient assessment.
5. Identify predisposing factors in the development of anxiety disorders.
6. Formulate nursing diagnoses and goals of care for patients with anxiety disorders.
7. Describe appropriate nursing interventions for behaviors associated with anxiety disorders.
8. Describe relevant criteria for evaluating nursing care of patients with anxiety disorders.
9. Discuss various modalities relevant to treatment of anxiety disorders.

KEY TERMS

agoraphobia	post-traumatic stress disorder
flooding	obsessive compulsive disorder
generalized anxiety disorder	ritualistic behavior
implosion therapy	simple phobia
panic disorder	social phobia
phobia	systematic desensitization

CHAPTER OUTLINE/LECTURE NOTES

I. Introduction
   A. Anxiety is a necessary force for survival. It is not the same as stress.
   B. Stress (or stressor) is an external pressure that is brought to bear upon the individual. Anxiety is the subjective emotional response to that stressor.
   C. Anxiety is distinguished from fear in that anxiety is an emotional process while fear is a cognitive one.
II. Historical Aspects
   A. Anxiety was once identified by its physiological symptoms, focusing largely on the cardiovascular system.
   B. Freud was the first to associate anxiety with neurotic behaviors.
   C. For many years, anxiety disorders were viewed as purely psychological or purely biological in nature.
III. Epidemiological Statistics
   A. Primary anxiety disorders represent one of the most prevalent mental health problems in the U.S. today.
   B. Anxiety disorders are more common in women than in men.
IV. How Much is Too Much?
   A. Anxiety is pathological if:
      1. The response is greatly disproportionate to the risk and severity of the danger or threat.
      2. The response continues beyond the existence of a potential danger or threat.

3. Intellectual, social, or occupational functioning is impaired.
4. The individual suffers from a psychosomatic effect (e.g., colitis or dermatitis).

V. Application of the Nursing Process
  A. Panic and generalized anxiety disorders: background assessment data
    1. Panic disorder
      a. Characterized by recurrent panic attacks, the onset of which are unpredictable, and manifested by intense apprehension, far, or terror, often associated with feelings of impending doom, and accompanied by intense physical discomfort.
        (1) dyspnea or smothering sensations
        (2) dizziness, unsteady feelings, or faintness
        (3) palpitations or tachycardia
        (4) trembling or shaking
        (5) sweating
        (6) choking
        (7) nausea or abdominal distress
        (8) depersonalization or derealization
        (9) numbness or paresthesias
        (10) hot flashes or chills
        (11) chest pain or discomfort
        (12) fear of dying
        (13) fear of going crazy or of doing something uncontrolled
      b. With agoraphobia
        (1) When panic disorder is accompanied by agoraphobia, the individual experiences the symptoms described above, but in addition, experiences a fear of being in places or situations from which escape might be difficult or embarrassing or in which help might not be available in the event of a panic attack.
    2. Generalized anxiety disorder
      a. Characterized by chronic, unrealistic, and excessive anxiety and worry. Symptoms include:
        (1) motor tension
        (2) Autonomic hyperactivity
        (3) Vigilance and scanning
    3. Predisposing factors to panic and generalized anxiety disorders
      a. Psychodynamic theory. An underdeveloped ego is not able to intervene when conflict occurs between the id and the superego, producing anxiety.
      b. Cognitive theory. This theory places emphasis on distorted cognition, which results in anxiety that is maintained by mistaken or dysfunctional appraisal of a situation.
      c. Biological aspects
        (1) Neuroanatomical. The lower brain centers may be responsible for initiating and controlling states of physiological arousal and for the involuntary homeostatic functions.
        (2) Biochemical. Abnormal elevations of blood lactate have been noted in patients with panic disorder.
        (3) Medical conditions. Various medical conditions, such as acute MI, hypoglycemia, mitral valve prolapse, and complex partial seizures, have been associated to a greater degree with individuals who suffer panic and generalized anxiety disorders than in the general population.
      d. Transactional model of stress-adaptation. The etiology of panic and generalized anxiety disorders is most likely influenced by multiple factors.
    4. Nursing diagnosis, planning/implementation
      a. Nursing intervention for the patient with panic or generalized anxiety disorder is aimed at relief of acute panic symptoms.
      b. The nurse also works on assisting the patient to take control of own life situation, and accept those situations over which he or she has no control.
    5. Evaluation is based on accomplishment of previously established outcome criteria.
  B. Phobias: background assessment data
    1. Agoraphobia without history of panic disorder. a fear of being in places or situations from which escape might be difficult, or in which help might not be available in the event of suddenly developing a panic or limited symptom attack.
    2. Social phobia. Characterized by a persistent fear of appearing shameful, stupid, or inept in the presence

of others.
3. Simple phobia. A persistent fear of a specific object or situation, other than the fear of being unable to escape from a situation or the fear of being humiliated in social situations.
4. Predisposing factors to phobias
   a. Psychoanalytic theory. Freud believed that during the oedipal period, the child becomes frightened of the aggression he fears the same sex parent feels for him. This fear is repressed, and displaced on to something safer, which becomes the phobic stimulus.
   b. Learning theory. Learning theorists believe that fears are learned, and they become conditioned responses when the individual escapes panic anxiety (a negative reinforcement) by avoiding the phobic stimulus.
   c. Cognitive theory. Cognitive theorists espouse that anxiety is the product of faulty cognitions or anxiety-including self-instructions.
   d. Biological aspects.
      (1) Temperament. Innate fears may represent a part of the overall characteristics or tendencies with which one is born that influence how he or she responds throughout life to specific situations.
   e. Life experiences. Certain early experiences may set the stage for phobic reactions later in life.
   f. Transactional model of stress-adaptation. The etiology of phobias is most likely influenced by multiple factors.
5. Nursing diagnosis, planning/implementation
   a. Nursing intervention for the patient with phobias is aimed at decreasing the fear and increasing the ability to function in the presence of the phobic stimulus.
6. Evaluation is based on accomplishment of previously established outcome criteria.
C. Obsessive compulsive disorder: background assessment data
1. Recurrent obsessions or compulsions sufficiently severe to cause marked distress, be time-consuming, or significantly interfere with the person's normal routine, occupational functioning, or usual social activities or relationships with others.
2. Predisposing factors to obsessive compulsive disorder.
   a. Psychoanalytic theory. Individuals with this disorder have weak, underdeveloped egos. Regression to the preoedipal phase of development during times of anxiety produce the symptoms of obsessions and compulsions.
   b. Learning theory. Obsessive compulsive behavior is viewed as a conditioned response to a traumatic event. The traumatic event produces anxiety and discomfort, and the individual learns to prevent it by avoiding the situation with which it is associated.
   c. Biological aspects.
      (1) Neuroanatomy. Lesions in various regions of the brain have been implicated in the neurobiology of obsessive compulsive disorder.
      (2) Physiology. Some individuals with obsessive compulsive disorder exhibit nonspecific EEG changes.
      (3) Biochemical. A decrease in the neurotransmitter serotonin may be influential in the etiology of obsessive compulsive disorder.
   d. Transactional model of stress-adaptation. The etiology of obsessive compulsive disorder is most likely influenced by multiple factors.
3. Nursing diagnosis, planning/implementation.
   a. Nursing intervention of the patient with obsessive compulsive disorder is aimed at helping him or her maintain anxiety at a manageable level without having to resort to use of ritualistic behavior. The focus is on development of more adaptive methods of coping with anxiety.
4. Evaluation is based on accomplishment of previously established outcome criteria.
D. Post-traumatic stress disorder (PTSD): background assessment data
1. The development of characteristic symptoms following a psychologically distressing event that is outside the range of usual human experience.
2. Symptoms may include a re-experiencing of the traumatic event, a sustained high level of anxiety/arousal, or a general numbing of responsiveness.
3. Predisposing factors to post-traumatic stress disorder.
   a. Psychosocial theory.
      (1) Seeks to explain why some individuals exposed to massive trauma develop PTSD while others do not.
      (2) Variables include characteristics that relate to the traumatic experience, the individual, and the

b. Learning theory. The avoidance behaviors and psychic numbing in response to a trauma are mediated by negative reinforcement (behaviors that decrease the emotional pain of the trauma).

c. Cognitive theory. Takes into consideration the cognitive appraisal of an event, and focuses on assumptions that an individual makes about the world.

d. Biological aspects. It is suggested that the symptoms related to the trauma are maintained by the production of endogenous opioid peptides that are produced in the face of arousal, and which result in increased feelings of comfort and control. When the stressor terminates, the individual may experience opioid withdrawal, the symptoms of which bear strong resemblance to those of PTSD.

e. Transactional model of stress-adaptation. The etiology of post-traumatic stress disorder is most likely influenced by multiple factors.

4. Nursing diagnosis, planning/implementation.

    a. Nursing intervention for the patient with PTSD is aimed at:

       (1) reassurance of safety.

       (2) decrease in maladaptive symptoms (e.g., flashbacks, nightmares).

       (3) demonstration of more adaptive coping strategies.

       (4) adaptive progression through the grief process.

5. Evaluation is based on accomplishment of previously established outcome criteria.

VI. Treatment Modalities for Anxiety Disorders

    A. Individual psychotherapy

    B. Cognitive therapy

    C. Behavior therapy

      1. Systematic desensitization

      2. Implosion therapy (flooding)

    D. Group/family therapy

    E. Psychopharmacology

VII. Summary

VIII. Review Questions

LEARNING ACTIVITY

BEHAVIORS ASSOCIATED WITH ANXIETY DISORDERS

Identify with which anxiety disorder the behaviors listed are associated. The first one is completed as an example.

a. Panic disorder
b. Agoraphobia
c. Simple phobia
d. Post-traumatic stress disorder

e. Generalized anxiety disorder
f. Social phobia
g. Obsessive compulsive disorder

___c___ 1. Janet becomes panicky when she gets near a dog.

_____ 2. Patricia weighs and measures her food. Long after everyone else has finished eating, she is still calculating the caloric value and remeasuring the amount.

_____ 3. Frances will not leave her home unless a friend or relative goes with her.

_____ 4. Harold has intrusive thoughts and sometimes visual illusions of his platoon's invasion of a village in Vietnam.

_____ 5. Sonja refuses to eat in a restaurant. She is afraid others will laugh at the way she eats.

_____ 6. About once a week, without warning, Stanley's heart begins to pound, he becomes short of breath, and sometimes he experiences chest pain. The doctor has ruled out physical problems.

_____ 7. Janie wants desperately to visit a foreign country with her friends, but because of her fear of needles, she has not been able to receive the required immunizations.

_____ 8. Helen is a very restless person. She is always nervous and keyed up. She worries about many things over which she has no control.

_____ 9. Timmie's family recently survived a tornado by taking refuge in the basement of their home. The home and all of its contents were destroyed. Timmie has nightmares about the event.

_____ 10. George never volunteers to speak in class. He is afraid his classmates will laugh at what he says.

_____ 11. Carl will go to church, but only if he can sit right near the door.

_____ 12. When Sally sees a spider on the floor, she screams and runs out of the room.

_____ 13. Every day when Wanda goes home from work, she cleans her house. She has told her friends not to call her during this time, and if anything interferes with her cleaning, she becomes very upset and starts over from the beginning.

_____ 14. Don has always been an excellent student and was valedictorian of his high school graduating class. Since starting college, he has been unusually worried about his academic performance. Lately, he has been unable to sleep, is irritable, has difficulty concentrating, and has begun experiencing nausea and vomiting due to worry that he will not do well academically.

_____ 15. Last month, on her way out of the hospital after working the evening shift, Amanda was abducted by man with a gun and taken to a remote area and raped. Since that time, she has become detached and estranged from her friends, she has difficulty sleeping, and has had problems concentrating at work.

TYPES OF
ANXIETY DISORDERS

PANIC DISORDER

GENERALIZED ANXIETY DISORDER

PHOBIAS

OBSESSIVE COMPULSIVE DISORDER

POST-TRAUMATIC
STRESS DISORDER

NURSING DIAGNOSES COMMON TO ANXIETY DISORDERS

PANIC AND GENERALIZED ANXIETY DISORDERS
    Anxiety (Panic)
    Powerlessness

PHOBIAS
    Fear
    Social Isolation

OBSESSIVE COMPULSIVE DISORDER
    Ineffective Individual Coping
    Altered Role Performance

POST-TRAUMATIC STRESS DISORDER
    Post-trauma Response
    Dysfunctional Grieving

TREATMENT MODALITIES
FOR
ANXIETY DISORDERS

INDIVIDUAL PSYCHOTHERAPY

COGNITIVE THERAPY

BEHAVIOR THERAPY
    Systematic Desensitization
    Implosion Therapy (Flooding)

GROUP/FAMILY THERAPY

PSYCHOPHARMACOLOGY

CHAPTER 21:   SOMATOFORM DISORDERS

CHAPTER FOCUS

The focus of this chapter is on nursing care of the patient with somatoform disorders. Predisposing factors and symptomatology are explored, and nursing care is presented in the context of the five steps of the nursing process. Medical treatment modalities are also discussed.

LEARNING OBJECTIVES

After reading this chapter, the student will be able to:

1.   Define the term "hysteria."
2.   Discuss historical aspects and epidemiological statistics related to somatoform disorders.
3.   Describe various types of somatoform disorders and identify symptomatology associated with each. Use this information in patient assessment.
4.   Identify predisposing factors in the development of somatoform disorders.
5.   Formulate nursing diagnoses and goals of care for patients with somatoform disorders.
6.   Describe appropriate nursing interventions for behaviors associated with somatoform disorders.
7.   Describe relevant criteria for evaluating nursing care of patients with somatoform disorders.
8.   Discuss various modalities relevant to treatment of somatoform disorders.

KEY TERMS

anosmia	primary gain
aphonia	pseudocyesis
hypochondriasis	secondary gain
hysteria	somatization
la belle indifference	tertiary gain

CHAPTER OUTLINE/LECTURE NOTES

I.   Introduction
   A. The somatoform disorders are characterized by physical symptoms suggesting medical disease, but no demonstrable organic pathology or known pathophysiological mechanism can be found to account for them.
   B. Somatization refers to all those mechanisms by which anxiety is translated into physical illness or bodily complaints.

II.   Historical Aspects
   A. The concept of hysteria, which is characterized by recurrent, multiple somatic complaints often described dramatically, is at least 4000 years old, and probably originated in Egypt.
   B. Witchcraft, demonology, and sorcery were associated with hysteria in the Middle Ages.
   C. In the 19th century, the French physician Paul Briquet attributed the disorder to dysfunction in the nervous system.
   D. Out of his work with hypnosis, Freud proposed that emotion which is not expressed can be "converted" into physical symptoms.

III.   Application of the Nursing Process
   A. Somatization disorder: background assessment data
      1. A chronic syndrome of multiple somatic symptoms that cannot be explained medically and are associated with psychological distress and long-term seeking of assistance from health care

professionals.

2. Any organ system may be affected, but common complaints involve the neurological, gastrointestinal, psychosexual, or cardiopulmonary systems.
3. Anxiety and depression are frequently manifested, and suicidal attempts and threats are not uncommon.
4. Predisposing factors to somatization disorder.
    a. Psychodynamic theory. Views somatoform disorders as the result of a poor mother-child relationship. When love is given conditionally, the child defends against insecurity by learning to gain affection and care through illness.
    b. Theory of family dynamics. In dysfunctional families, when a child becomes ill, a shift in focus is made from the open conflict to the child's illness, leaving unresolved the underlying issues which the family is unable to confront in open manner. Somatization brings some stability to the family, and positive reinforcement to the child.
    c. Cultural and environmental factors. Various cultures deal with physical symptoms in different ways. Environmental factors may be influential when there is a lack of language sophistication required to express oneself psychologically or social restrictions against conceptualizing life difficulties in psychological terminology.
    d. Genetic factors. No genetic link can be made to somatoform disorders, although some studies have shown it is more prevalent in some families than others.
    e. Transactional model of stress-adaptation. The etiology of somatization disorder is most likely influenced by multiple factors.
5. Nursing diagnoses, planning/implementation.
    a. Nursing intervention for the patient with somatization disorder is aimed at assisting the patient to learn to cope with stress by means other than preoccupation with physical symptoms.
    b. The nurse also works to help the patient correlate appearance of the physical symptoms with times of stress.
6. Evaluation is based on accomplishment of previously established outcome criteria.

B. Somatoform pain disorder: background assessment data
1. The predominant disturbance in somatoform pain disorder is severe and prolonged pain for which there is no adequate medical explanation.
2. Even when organic pathology is detected, the pain complaint may be evidenced by the correlation of a stressful situation with the onset of the symptom.
3. The disorder may be maintained by:
    a. Primary gains: the symptom enables the patient to avoid some unpleasant activity.
    b. Secondary gains: the symptom promotes emotional support or attention for the patient.
    c. Tertiary gains: in dysfunctional families, the physical symptom may take such a position that the real issue is disregarded and remains unresolved, even though some of the conflict is relieved.
4. Predisposing factors to somatoform pain disorder.
    a. Psychoanalytic theory. Theorizes that pain for some patients serve the purposes of punishment and atonement for unconscious guilt. Occurs with individuals who have been severely punished as children.
    b. Behavioral theory. In behavioral terminology, psychogenic pain is explained as a response that is learned through operant and classical conditioning. Occurs when pain behaviors are positive or negatively reinforced.
    c. Theory of family dynamics. "Pain games" may be played in families burdened by conflict. Pain may be used for manipulating and gaining the advantage in interpersonal relationships. Tertiary gain may also be influential.
    d. Neurophysiological theory. Postulates that the cerebral cortex is involved in inhibiting the firing of afferent pain fibers. These individuals may have decreased levels of serotonin and endorphins.
    e. Transactional model of stress-adaptation. The etiology of somatoform pain disorder is most likely influenced by multiple factors.
5. Nursing diagnosis, planning/implementation
    a. Nursing intervention for the patient with somatoform pain disorder is aimed at relief from pain.
    b. Emphasis is placed on learning more adaptive coping strategies for dealing with stress. Reinforcement is given at times when the patient is not focusing on pain.
6. Evaluation is based on accomplishments of previously established outcome criteria.

C. Hypochondriasis: background assessment data
1. Unrealistic preoccupation with fear of having a serious illness.

2. Even in the presence of medical disease, the symptoms are grossly disproportionate to the degree of pathology.
3. Predisposing factors to hypochondriasis
   a. Psychodynamic theory
      (1) One view suggests that hypochondriasis is an ego defense mechanism. Physical complaints are the expression of low self-esteem and feelings of worthlessness, as it is easier to feel something is wrong with the body than to feel something is wrong with the self.
      (2) Another psychodynamic view explains hypochondriasis as the transformation of aggressive and hostile wishes toward others into physical complaints to others.
      (3) Still other psychodynamicists have viewed hypochondriasis as a defense against guilt.
   b. Cognitive theory. Cognitive theorists view hypochondriasis as arising out of perceptual and cognitive abnormalities.
   c. Sociocultural/familial factors. Somatic complaints are often reinforced when the sick role serves to relieve the individual from the need to deal with a stressful situation, whether it be within society or within the family constellation.
   d. Past experience with physical illness. Personal experience, or the experience of close family members, with serious or life-threatening illness can predispose an individual to hypochondriasis.
   e. Genetic influences. Little is known about hereditary influences with hypochondriasis.
   f. Transactional model of stress-adaptation. The etiology of hypochondriasis is most likely influenced by multiple factors.
4. Nursing diagnosis, planning/implementation
   a. Nursing intervention for the patient with hypochondriasis is aimed at relieving the fear of serious illness.
   b. The focus is on decreasing the preoccupation with and unrealistic interpretation of bodily signs and sensations.
   c. The nurse also works to help the patient increase feelings of self-worth and resolve internalized anger.
5. Evaluation is based on accomplishment of previously established outcome criteria.
D. Conversion Disorder
1. A loss of, or change in, bodily functioning resulting from a psychological conflict, the bodily symptoms of which cannot be explained by any known medical disorder or pathophysiological mechanism.
2. The most obvious and "classic" conversion symptoms are those that suggest neurologic disease, and occur following a situation that produces extreme psychological stress for the individual.
3. The person often expresses a relative lack of concern that is out of keeping with the severity of the impairment. This lack of concern is identified as *la belle indifference* and may be a clue to the physician that the problem is psychological rather than physical.
4. Predisposing factors to conversion disorder
   a. Psychoanalytic theory. Emotions associated with a traumatic event that the individual cannot express because of moral or ethical unacceptability are "converted" into physical symptoms. The symptom is symbolic in some way of the original emotional trauma.
   b. Theory of interpersonal communication. Conversion symptoms are viewed as a type of nonverbal communication. With physical symptoms, the individual communicates that he or she (or the relationship) needs special treatment or consideration.
   c. Neurophysiological theory. Suggests that some patients with conversion disorder have a diminishment in central nervous system arousal.
   d. Behavioral theory. Suggests that conversion symptoms are learned through positive reinforcement from cultural, social, and interpersonal influences.
   e. Transactional model of stress-adaptation. The etiology of conversion disorder is most likely influenced by multiple factors.
5. Nursing diagnosis, planning/implementation
   a. Nursing intervention for the patient with conversion disorder is aimed at recovery of the lost or altered function.
   b. Emphasis is given to assisting the patient with activities of daily living until the function is regained. Care is given not to reinforce the physical limitation.
E. Body dysmorphic disorder: background assessment data
1. Characterized by the exaggerated belief that the body is deformed or defective in some specific way.
2. Symptoms of depression and characteristics associated with obsessive compulsive personality are

common.
    3. Has been closely associated with delusional thinking, and in Europe, it is considered to be a psychosis.
    4. Predisposing factors to body dysmorphic disorder
       a. Etiology is unknown, but presumed to be psychologic.
       b. Predisposing factors may be similar to those associated with hypochondriasis or phobias.
       c. It is most likely that multiple factors are involved in the predisposition to body dysmorphic disorder.
    5. Nursing diagnosis, planning/implementation
       a. Nursing intervention for the patient with body dysmorphic disorder is aimed at development of a realistic perception of body appearance.
       b. A focus is on resolution of repressed fears and anxieties that contribute to altered body image.
       c. Positive reinforcement is given for accomplishments unrelated to physical appearance.
    6. Evaluation is based on accomplishment of previously established outcome criteria.
IV.   Treatment Modalities
    A. Individual psychotherapy
    B. Group psychotherapy
    C. Behavior therapy
    D. Psychopharmacology
V.   Summary
VII.   Review Questions

LEARNING ACTIVITY

BEHAVIORS ASSOCIATED WITH SOMATOFORM DISORDERS

Identify with which somatoform disorder the behaviors listed are associated. List the primary nursing diagnosis for each.

- a. Somatization Disorder
- b. Somatoform Pain Disorder
- c. Hypochondriasis
- d. Conversion Disorder
- e. Body Dysmorphic Disorder

_____ 1. Nancy fell on the ice last winter and injured her elbow. She complains that she has had pain ever since, even though x-rays reveal the elbow has healed appropriately.

Nursing diagnosis:_____

_____ 2. Virginia has some freckles across her nose and cheeks. She visits dermatologists regularly trying to find one who will "get rid of these huge spots on my skin."

Nursing diagnosis:_____

_____ 3. Franklin is assigned to secure a contract for his company. The boss tells Franklin, "If we don't get this contract, the company may have to fold." When Franklin wakes up on the morning of the negotiations, he is unable to see. The doctor has ruled out organic pathology.

Nursing diagnosis:_____

_____ 4. Sarah has had what she calls a "delicate stomach" for years. She has sought out many physicians with complaints of nausea and vomiting, abdominal pain, bloating, and diarrhea. No organic pathology can be detected.

Nursing diagnosis:_____

_____ 5. John's father died of a massive myocardial infarction when John (now age 34) was 15 years old. The two of them were playing basketball at the time. Since then, John becomes panicky when he feels his heart beating faster than usual. He takes his pulse several times a day, and seeks out a physical exam from his physician several times a year.

Nursing diagnosis:_____

TYPES OF SOMATIZATION DISORERS

Somatization Disorder

Somatoform Pain Disorder

Hypochondriasis

Conversion Disorder

Body Dysmorphic Disorder

NURSING DIAGNOSES COMMON TO SOMATOFORM DISORDERS

SOMATIZATION DISORDER
Ineffective individual coping
Knowledge deficit (psychological causes for
physical symptoms)

SOMATOFORM PAIN DISORDER
Chronic pain
Social isolation

HYPOCHONDRIASIS
Fear (of having serious illness)
Self-esteem disturbance

CONVERSION DISORDER
Sensory-perceptual alteration
Self-care deficit

BODY DYSMORPHIC DISORDER
Body image disturbance

TREATMENT MODALITIES
FOR
SOMATOFORM DISORDERS

Individual Psychotherapy

Group Psychotherapy

Behavior Therapy

Psychopharmacology

CHAPTER 22: DISSOCIATIVE DISORDERS

CHAPTER FOCUS

The focus of this chapter is on nursing care of the patient with dissociative disorders. Predisposing factors and symptomatology are explored, and nursing care is presented in the context of the five steps of the nursing process. Medical treatment modalities are also discussed.

LEARNING OBJECTIVES

After reading this chapter, the student will be able to:

1. Discuss historical aspects and epidemiological statistics related to dissociative disorders.
2. Describe various types of dissociative disorders and identify symptomatology associated with each. Utilize this information in patient assessment.
3. Identify predisposing factors in the development of dissociative disorders.
4. Formulate nursing diagnoses and goals of care for patients with dissociative disorders.
5. Describe appropriate nursing interventions for behaviors associated with dissociative disorders.
6. Describe relevant criteria for evaluating nursing care of patients with dissociative disorders.
7. Discuss various modalities relevant to treatment of dissociative disorders.

KEY TERMS

abreaction	derealization
amnesia	fugue
association	generalized amnesia
directed	hypnosis
free	integration
continuous amnesia	localized amnesia
depersonalization	selected amnesia

CHAPTER OUTLINE/LECTURE NOTES

I. Introduction
    A. The essential feature of dissociative disorders is a disturbance or alteration in the normally integrative functions of identity, memory, or consciousness.
    B. Dissociative responses occur when anxiety becomes overwhelming and a disorganization of the personality ensues.
    C. Four types of dissociative disorders include psychogenic amnesia, psychogenic fugue, multiple personality, and depersonalization disorder.
II. Historical Aspects
    A. The concept of dissociation was first formulated during the 19th century.
    B. Freud viewed dissociation as a type of repression, an active defense mechanism utilized in the removal of threatening or unacceptable mental contents from conscious awareness.
III. Epidemiological Statistics
    A. Dissociative syndromes are statistically quite rare.
    B. Psychogenic amnesia and psychogenic fugue are both rare, but occur most often under conditions of war or during natural disasters or other severe psychosocial stress.

commonly begins in childhood, but symptoms do not appear until adolescence or early adulthood.

    D. The prevalence of severe depersonalization disorder is unknown. Single brief episodes appear to be common in young adulthood, particularly in time of severe stress.

IV. Application of the Nursing Process

    A. Psychogenic amnesia: background assessment data

        1. Defined as sudden inability to recall important personal information that is too extensive to be explained by ordinary forgetfulness, and which is not due to an organic mental disorder, including states of drug intoxication and withdrawal.

        2. Four types of disturbance in recall:

            a. Localized amnesia. The inability to recall all incidents associated with the traumatic event for a specific time period following the event (usually a few hours to a few days).

            b. Selective amnesia. The inability to recall only certain incidents associated with a traumatic event for a specific time period following the event.

            c. Generalized amnesia. The inability to recall anything that has happened during the individual's entire lifetime, including personal identity.

            d. Continuous amnesia. The inability to recall events occurring after a specific time up to and including the present.

        3. Predisposing factors to psychogenic amnesia

            a. Psychodynamic theory. Freud described amnesia as the result of repression of distressing mental contents from conscious awareness.

            b. Behavioral theory. Suggests that psychogenic amnesia may be the result of learning and reinforced by primary and secondary gains for the individual.

            c. Biological theory. Some efforts have been made to explain psychogenic amnesia on the basis of neurophysiologic dysfunction, although current information is inadequate and lacking in credibility.

            d. Transactional model of stress-adaptation. The etiology of psychogenic amnesia is most likely influenced by multiple factors.

        4. Nursing diagnosis, planning/implementation

            a. Nursing intervention for the patient with psychogenic amnesia is aimed at ability to recall lost mental contents.

            b. The nurse also works at assisting the patient to deal more appropriately with severe anxiety.

        5. Evaluation is based on accomplishment of previously established outcome criteria.

    B. Psychogenic fugue: background assessment data

        1. The characteristic feature of psychogenic fugue is a sudden, unexpected travel away from home or customary workplace.

        2. An individual in a fugue state is unable to recall personal identity, and assumption of a new identity is common.

        3. Predisposing factors to psychogenic fugue

            a. Psychodynamic theory, behavioral theory and possible biological theory. Same as psychogenic amnesia.

            b. Theory of family dynamics. Unsatisfactory parent/child relationship, with subsequent internalization of loss, has been implicated in the etiology of psychogenic fugue. Unfulfilled separation anxiety, a defect in personality development, and unmet dependency needs may also be related to dysfunctional family dynamics.

            c. Transactional model of stress-adaptation. The etiology of psychogenic fugue is most likely influenced by multiple factors.

        4. Nursing diagnosis, planning/implementation

            a. Nursing intervention for the patient with psychogenic fugue is aimed at protection of patient and others from uncontrolled aggression.

            b. The nurse also works at assisting the patient to deal more appropriately with severe anxiety.

        5. Evaluation is based on accomplishment of previously established outcome criteria.

    C. Multiple personality disorder: background assessment data

        1. Characterized by the existence of two or more personalities within a single individual.

        2. The transition from one personality to another is usually sudden, often dramatic, and usually precipitated by stress.

        3. Predisposing factors to multiple personality disorder.

            a. Biologic theories.

               (1) Genetics. Multiple personality disorder is more common in first degree biological relatives of

(1) Genetics. Multiple personality disorder is more common in first degree biological relatives of people with the disorder than in the general population.

(2) Organic. Various studies have suggested a possible link to certain neurological alterations (e.g., temporal lobe epilepsy, severe migraine headaches, and cerebral cortical damage) and multiple personality disorder.

    b. Psychological influences. A growing body of evidence points to the etiology of MPD as a set of traumatic experiences that overwhelms the individual's capacity to cope by any means other than dissociation. These experiences usually take the form of severe physical, sexual or psychological abuse by a parent or significant other in the child's life.

    c. Theory of family dynamics. A dysfunctional family system, with at least one caretaker who exhibits severe psychopathology, has been implicated as an etiology of MPD.

    d. Transactional model of stress-adaptation. The etiology of multiple personality disorder is most likely influenced by multiple factors.

  4. Nursing diagnosis, planning/implementation

    a. Nursing intervention for the patient with multiple personality disorder is aimed at protection from self-directed violence.

    b. The nurse also works at assisting the patient to understand the reasons for existence of various personalities and the importance of eventual integration of the personalities into one.

  5. Evaluation is based on accomplishment of previously established outcome criteria.

D. Depersonalization disorder: background assessment data

  1. Characterized by a temporary change in the quality of self-awareness, which often takes the form of feelings of unreality, changes in body image, feelings of detachment from the environment, or a sense of observing oneself from outside the body.

  2. Depersonalization is defined as a disturbance in the perception of oneself.

  3. Derealization is described as an alteration in the perception of the external environment.

  4. Symptoms of depersonalization disorder are often accompanied by anxiety, dizziness, fear of going insane, depression, obsessive thoughts, somatic complaints, and a disturbance in the subjective sense of time.

  5. Predisposing factors to depersonalization disorder.

    a. Physiological theories. Suggest that the phenomenon of depersonalization has a neurophysiologic basis, such as brain tumor or epilepsy.

    b. Psychodynamic theories. Place emphasis on psychic conflict and disturbances of ego structure in the predisposition to depersonalization disorder.

    c. Transactional model of stress-adaptation. The etiology of depersonalization disorder is most likely influenced by multiple factors.

  6. Nursing diagnosis, planning/implementation

    a. Nursing intervention for the patient with depersonalization disorder is aimed at promoting accurate perception of self and the environment.

    b. The nurse also works at assisting the patient to respond more adaptively to severe anxiety.

  7. Evaluation is based on accomplishment of previously established outcome criteria.

V. Treatment Modalities

A. Psychogenic amnesia

  1. Most cases resolve spontaneously.

  2. Refractory conditions may require intravenous administration of amobarbital in the retrieval of lost memories.

  3. Supportive psychotherapy may also be useful.

  4. Hypnosis has been used successfully.

B. Psychogenic fugue

  1. Recovery is usually rapid, spontaneous, and complete.

  2. Supportive care may be required.

  3. Refractory conditions may require encouragement, persuasion, or directed association, either alone, or in combination with hypnosis or amobarbital administration.

C. Multiple personality disorder

  1. Integration is considered desirable, but in some cases a reasonable degree of conflict-free collaboration among the personalities is al that can be achieved.

  2. Long-term psychotherapy, with the use of abreaction, has been successful.

  3. Hypnosis is usually used in the process of integration.

D. Depersonalization disorder

1. No particular therapy has proven widely successful.
2. Pharmacotherapy with dextroamphetamines or amobarbital has been tried with inconclusive results.
3. Benzodiazepines provide symptomatic relief if anxiety is an important element of the clinical condition.
4. Some clinicians believe long-term psychoanalysis may be helpful for patients with intrapsychic conflict.

VI. Summary
VII. Review Questions

LEARNING ACTIVITY

BEHAVIORS ASSOCIATED WITH DISSOCIATIVE DISORDERS

Identify with which dissociative disorder the behaviors listed are associated. List the primary nursing diagnosis for each.

a. Localized amnesia
b. Selective amnesia
c. Generalized amnesia
d. Continuous amnesia

e. Psychogenic fugue
f. Multiple Personality Disorder
g. Depersonalization Disorder

_____ 1. A young man is brought into the emergency department by the police. He does not know who he is or anything at all about his life.

_____ 2. A young man is brought into the emergency department by the police. He gives his identity and home address (which is several hundred miles away) to the admissions clerk. He tells the nurse he is very frightened, because he doesn't know when or how he came to be in this place.

_____ 3. Sandra is a clerk in an all-night convenience store. Three nights ago, the store was robbed at gunpoint, and Sandra was locked in a storage compartment for several hours until the manager was contacted by passersby who reported the robbery. She has been unable to recall the incident until just today, when details began to emerge. She is now able to report the entire event to the authorities.

_____ 4. Sam is a salesman for a leading manufacturing company. His job requires that he make presentations for large corporations that are considering Sam's company's product. Sam is up for promotion, and realizes that the outcome of these presentations will weigh heavily on whether or not he gets the promotion. Lately, he has been worried that he is going insane. Each time he is about to make a presentation, his thinking becomes "foggy," his body feels lifeless, and he describes the feeling as being somewhat "anesthetized." These episodes sometimes last for hours, and are beginning to interfere with his performance.

_____ 5. Melody's husband complained of severe chest pain. Melody called the ambulance and accompanied her husband to the hospital. He died of a massive myocardial infarction in the emergency department. With the help of family and friends, Melody made arrangements for the memorial service and the burial. Now that it is all over, Melody is able to remember only certain aspects about the time since her husband first experienced the severe pain. She remembers the doctor telling her that her husband was dead, but she cannot remember attending the funeral service.

_____ 6. Margaret explains to the nurse that during the last year, she has periods of time for which she cannot account. She has been attending college, and she finds pages of notes in her notebook that she cannot recall writing. Her roommate recently recounted an incident that took place when they were supposedly out together, for which Margaret has no recall. Most recently she has been hospitalized when her roommate found her unconscious in their room with an empty bottle of sleeping pills beside her. She tells the nurse she has no memory of taking the pills.

_____ 7. Kelly was involved in an automobile accident in which her best friend was killed. Kelly remembers nothing about the accident, nor does she remember anything that has occurred since the accident.

TYPES OF DISSOCIATIVE DISORDERS

Psychogenic Amnesia

Psychogenic Fugue

Multiple Personality

Depersonalization Disorder

NURSING DIAGNOSES COMMON TO DISSOCIATIVE DISORDERS

PSYCHOGENIC AMNESIA
>Altered thought processes
>Powerlessness

PSYCHOGENIC FUGUE
>High risk for violence directed toward others
>Ineffective individual coping

MULTIPLE PERSONALITY DISORDER
>High risk for self-directed violence
>Personal identity disturbance

DEPERSONALIZATION DISORDER
>Sensory-perceptual alteration (visual and
>   kinesthetic)
>Anxiety (severe to panic)

TREATMENT MODALITIES FOR DISSOCIATIVE DISORDERS

PSYCHOGENIC AMNESIA
1. Time and removal of the stressor
2. Amobarbital
3. Supportive psychotherapy
4. Hypnosis

PSYCHOGENIC FUGUE
1. Time and removal of the stressor
2. Supportive care
3. Hypnosis or amobarbital

MULTIPLE PERSONALITY DISORDER
1. Integration of the personalities
2. Long-term psychotherapy with abreaction
3. Hypnosis

DEPERSONALIZATION DISORDER
1. Psychopharmacology
2. Long-term psychoanalysis

CHAPTER 23:   SEXUAL DISORDERS

CHAPTER FOCUS

The focus of this chapter is on nursing care of the patient with sexual disorders.   Predisposing factors and symptomatology are explored, and nursing care is presented in the context of the five steps of the nursing process. Medical treatment modalities are also discussed.

LEARNING OBJECTIVES

After reading this chapter, the student will be able to:

1.   Describe developmental processes associated with human sexuality.
2.   Discuss historical and epidemiological aspects of paraphilias.
3.   Identify various types of paraphilias.
4.   Discuss predisposing factors associated with the etiology of paraphilias.
5.   Describe the physiology of the human sexual response.
6.   Discuss historical and epidemiological aspects of sexual dysfunction.
7.   Identify various types of sexual dysfunction.
8.   Discuss predisposing factors associated with the etiology of sexual dysfunction.
9.   Conduct a sexual history.
10.   Formulate nursing diagnoses and goals of care for patients with sexual disorders.
11.   Describe appropriate nursing interventions for patients with sexual disorders.
12.   Describe relevant criteria for evaluating nursing care of patients with sexual disorders.
13.   Identify various treatment modalities for patients with sexual disorders.
14.   Discuss alternative sexual life styles.
15.   Identify various types of sexually transmitted diseases and discuss the consequences of each.

KEY TERMS

anorgasmia	pedophilia
dyspareunia	premature ejaculation
exhibitionism	retarded ejaculation
fetishism	sadism
frotteurism	sensate focus
gonorrhea	syphilis
homosexuality	transsexualism
lesbianism	transvestic fetishism
masochism	vaginismus
orgasm	voyeurism
paraphilia	

CHAPTER OUTLINE/LECTURE NOTES

I.   Introduction
    A. Sexuality is a basic need and an aspect of humanness that cannot be separated from life events.
    B. Although not all nurses need to be educated as sex therapists, they can readily integrate information on sexuality in the care they give by focusing on preventive, therapeutic, and educational interventions to assist individuals attain, regain, or maintain sexual health.
II.   Development of Human Sexuality

A. Birth through age 12
   1. By age 2 or 1-1/2, children know what gender they are.
   2. By age 4 or 5, children engage in heterosexual play.
   3. Late childhood and preadolescence may be characterized by homosexual play.
   4. Ages 10 to 12 are preoccupied with pubertal changes and the beginnings of romantic interest in the opposite gender.
B. Adolescence
   1. Adolescents relate to sexual issues such as how to deal with new or more powerful sexual feelings, whether to participate in various types of sexual behavior, how to recognize love, how to prevent unwanted pregnancy, and how to define age-appropriate sex roles.
C. Adulthood. This period begins at approximately 20 years of age and continues to age 65.
   1. Marital sex. Choosing a marital partner or developing a sexual relationship with another individual is one of the major tasks in the early years of this life cycle stage.
   2. Extramarital sex. Approximately one-half of all married men have extramarital sex at some time in their lives, compared with about one-quarter of all women.
   3. Sex and the single person. Attitudes about sexual intimacy vary greatly from individual to individual. Some enjoy their freedom and independence, while others are desperately seeking an intimate relationship.
   4. The middle years--46 to 65. Hormonal changes occurring during this period produce changes in sexual activity for both men and women.
III. Sexual Disorders
A. Paraphilias - a term used to identify repetitive or preferred sexual fantasies or behaviors that involve the preference for use of a nonhuman object, repetitive sexual activity with humans involving real or simulated suffering or humiliation, and repetitive sexual activity with nonconsenting partners.
   1. Historical aspects
      a. At certain times in history, various sexual behaviors have been, and still are, condemned by certain social and religious sanctions.
   2. Epidemiological statistics
      a. Most paraphiliacs are men, and over 50% of these individuals develop the onset of their paraphilic arousal prior to age 18.
   3. Types of paraphilias
      a. Exhibitionism - characterized by recurrent, intense, sexual urges and sexually arousing fantasies involving the exposure of one's genitals to a stranger.
      b. Fetishism - involves recurrent, intense, sexual urges and sexually arousing fantasies involving the use of nonliving objects (e.g., bras, underpants, stockings).
      c. Frotteurism - the recurrent preoccupation with intense sexual urges or fantasies involving touching or rubbing against a nonconsenting person.
      d. Pedophilia - recurrent sexual urges and sexually arousing fantasies involving sexual activity with a prepubescent child.
      e. Sexual masochism - recurrent, intense, sexual urges and sexually arousing fantasies involving the act (real, not simulated) of being humiliated, beaten, bound, or otherwise made to suffer.
      f. Sexual sadism - recurrent, intense, sexual urges and sexually arousing fantasies involving acts (real, not simulated) in which the psychological or physical suffering (including humiliation) of the victim is sexually exciting.
      g. Voyeurism - recurrent, intense, sexual urges and sexually arousing fantasies involving the act of observing unsuspecting people, usually strangers, who are either naked, in the process of disrobing, or engaging in sexual activity.
   4. Predisposing factors to paraphilias
      a. Biological factors. Various studies have implicated several organic factors in the etiology of paraphilias. These include abnormalities in the limbic system and the temporal lobe. Abnormal levels of androgens have also been implicated.
      b. Psychoanalytic theory. Suggests that a paraphiliac is one who has failed the normal developmental process toward heterosexual adjustment. This occurs when the individual fails to resolve the oedipal crisis and either identifies with the parent of the opposite gender or selects an inappropriate object for libido cathexis.
      c. Behavioral theory. The behavioral model hypothesizes that whether or not an individual engages in paraphiliac behavior depends on the type of reinforcement he receives following the behavior. The initial act may be committed for various reason (e.g., modeling the paraphilic behavior of others,

mimicking sexual behavior depicted in the media). But once the initial act has been committed, a conscious evaluation of the behavior occurs, and a choice is made of whether or not to repeat it.

    d. Transactional model of stress-adaptation. It is most likely that the etiology of paraphilias is influenced by multiple factors.

  5. Treatment modalities

    a. Biologic treatment. The focus of this treatment is on blocking or decreasing the level of circulating androgens.

    b. Psychoanalytic therapy. With this type of therapy, the patient is assisted to identify unresolved conflicts and traumas from early childhood, thus resolving the anxiety that prevents him or her from forming appropriate sexual relationships.

    c. Behavior therapy. Aversion techniques, such as the use of electric shock and chemical induction of nausea and vomiting, usually in combination with exposure to photographs depicting the undesired behavior, have been used to modify undesirable paraphilic behavior.

  6. Role of the nurse

    a. Nursing may best become involved in the primary prevention process.

    b. The focus of primary prevention in sexual disorders is to intervene in home life or other facets of childhood in an effort to prevent problems from developing.

    c. An additional concern of primary prevention is to assist in the development of adaptive coping strategies to deal with stressful life situations.

B. Sexual dysfunctions

  1. Usually occur as a problem in one of the following phases of the sexual response cycle:

    a. Phase I: Appetitive

    b. Phase II: Excitement

    c. Phase III: Plateau

    d. Phase IV: Orgasm

    e. Phase V: Resolution

  2. Historical and epidemiological aspects related to sexual dysfunction

    a. Concurrent with the cultural changes occurring during the sexual revolution of the 1960's and 1970's came an increase in scientific research into sexual physiology and sexual dysfunctions.

    b. Masters and Johnson pioneered this work with their studies on human sexual response and the treatment of sexual dysfunctions.

  3. Types of sexual dysfunction

    a. Sexual desire disorders

      (1) Hypoactive sexual desire disorder. Persistent or recurrent deficiency or absence of sexual fantasies and desire for sexual activity.

      (2) Sexual aversion disorder. Persistent or recurrent extreme aversion to, and avoidance of, all or almost all genital sexual contact with a sexual partner.

    b. Sexual arousal disorders

      (1) Female sexual arousal disorder. Failure to attain or maintain the lubrication-swelling response, or experience a subjective sense of sexual excitement and pleasure in a female during sexual activity.

      (2) Male sexual arousal disorder. Inability to attain or maintain erection, or experience a subjective sense of sexual excitement and pleasure in a male during sexual activity.

    c. Orgasm disorders

      (1) Inhibited female orgasm (anorgasmia). The recurrent and persistent inhibition of the female orgasm, as manifested by the absence or delay of orgasm following a period of sexual excitement judged adequate in intensity and duration to produce such a response.

      (2) Inhibited male orgasm (retarded ejaculation). Inability to ejaculate, even though the man has a firm erection and has had more than adequate stimulation.

      (3) Premature ejaculation. Persistent or recurrent ejaculation with minimal sexual stimulation or before, upon, or shortly after penetration and before the person wishes it.

    d. Sexual pain disorders

      (1) Dyspareunia. Recurrent or persistent genital pain in either a male or female before, during or after sexual intercourse, that is not associated with vaginismus or with lack of lubrication.

      (2) Vaginismus. An involuntary constriction of the outer one-third of the vagina that prevents penile insertion and intercourse.

  4. Predisposing factors to sexual dysfunctions

a. Biological factors. Suggestive evidence exists of a relationship between serum testosterone and hypoactive sexual desire disorder in men and increased libido in women. Certain medications, such as antihypertensives, antipsychotics, antidepressants, anxiolytics, and anticonvulsants may also be implicated in the etiology of hypoactive sexual desire disorder. Erectile disorders in men may be affected by arteriosclerosis and diabetes. In women, consumption of alcohol, as well as certain medications, have been shown to affect a woman's ability to have orgasms.

b. Psychosocial factors. A number of psychosocial factors have been associated with sexual desire disorders, as well as with virtually all the sexual disorders.

c. Transactional model of stress-adaptation. The etiology of sexual disorders is mostly likely influenced by multiple factors.

IV. Application of the Nursing Process
   A. Assessment. A tool for gathering a sexual history is included. Additional information should be gathered for the patients who have medical or surgical conditions that may affect their sexuality; patients with infertility problems, sexually transmitted disease, or complaints of sexual inadequacy; patients who are pregnant, or present with gynecologic problems; those seeking information on abortion or family planning; and individuals in premarital, marital, and psychiatric counseling.
   B. Nursing diagnoses, planning/implementation
      1. Nursing intervention for the patient with sexual disorders is aimed at assisting the individual to gain or regain the aspect of his or her sexuality that is desired.
      2. The nurse must remain nonjudgmental and ensure that personal feelings, attitudes, and values have been clarified and do not interfere with acceptance of the patient.
   C. Evaluation is based on accomplishment of previously established outcome criteria.

V. Treatment Modalities. Various sexual dysfunctions and some treatment modalities that have been tried are listed here.
   A. Hypoactive sexual desire disorder
      1. Testosterone
      2. Cognitive therapy
      3. Behavioral therapy
      4. Marital therapy
   B. Sexual aversion disorder
      1. Systematic desensitization
      2. Antidepressant medications
   C. Female sexual arousal disorder
      1. Sensate focus exercises
   D. Male erectile disorder
      1. Sensate focus exercises
      2. Group therapy
      3. Hypnotherapy
      4. Systematic desensitization
      5. Testosterone
      6. Penile implantation
   E. Inhibited male or female orgasm
      1. Sensate focus exercises
      2. Directed masturbation training
   F Premature ejaculation
      1. Sensate focus exercises
      2. "Squeeze" technique
   G. Dyspareunia
      1. Physical and gynecologic examination
      2. Systematic desensitization
   H. Vaginismus
      1. Education of the woman and her partner regarding the anatomy and physiology of the disorder.
      2. Systematic desensitization with dilators of graduated sizes.

VI. Alternative Sexual Life Styles
   A. Homosexuality - the life style that expresses a sexual preference for individuals of the same gender. This is only seen by the psychiatric community as a problem when the individual experiences "persistent and marked distress about his or her sexual orientation."

1. Predisposing factors
    a. Biological theories. It has been suggested that a genetic tendency for homosexuality may be inherited, or that a decreased level of testosterone may be influential. Neither hypothesis has been substantiated.
    b. Psychosocial theories.
        (1) Freud suggested a possible fixation in the stage of development where homosexual tendencies are common.
        (2) Bieber suggested a dysfunctional family pattern as an etiological influence in the development of male homosexuality. The mother was described as dominant, overprotective, possessive, and seductive in her interactions with her son. The father was found to be passive, distant, and covertly or overtly hostile, and was openly devalued and dominated by the mother.
2. Special concerns
    a. Sexually transmitted diseases, in particular, AIDS.
    b. Discovery of their sexual orientation.
    c. Fear of being rejected by parents and significant others.
    d. Discrimination within society.
B. Transsexualism - a disorder of gender identity or gender dysphoria (unhappiness or dissatisfaction with one's gender) of the most extreme variety. An individual, despite having the anatomical characteristics of a given gender, has the self-perception of being of the opposite gender.
    1. Predisposing factors
        a. Biologic theories. There has been some speculation that gender-disordered individuals may be exposed to inappropriate hormones during the prenatal period, which can result in a genetic female having male genitals, or a genetic male having female genitals. Evidence is inconclusive.
        b. Psychosocial theories
            (1) Extensive, pervasive childhood femininity in a boy or childhood masculinity in a girl increases the likelihood of transsexualism.
            (2) Repeated cross-dressing of a young adult.
            (3) Lack of separation/individuation of a boy from his mother.
    2. Special concerns
        a. Extensive psychological testing prior to surgical intervention.
        b. Hormonal treatment initiated during this period.
        c. Both males and females continue to receive maintenance hormone therapy following surgery.
C. Bisexuality - an individual who is not exclusively heterosexual or homosexual, but engages in sexual activity with members of both genders.
    1. Predisposing factors
        a. Little research exists on the etiology of bisexuality.
        b. Freud believed that all humans are inherently bisexual.
        c. Riddle suggests that gender identity (determining whether one is male or female) seems to be established during the preschool years.
        d. Sexual identity (determining whether one is heterosexual or homosexual or both) most likely continues to evolve throughout one's lifetime.
VII. Sexually Transmitted Diseases
    A. Sexually transmitted diseases (STDs) are a group of disease syndromes that can be transmitted sexually irrespective of whether the disease has genital pathologic manifestations. They may be transmitted from one person to another through heterosexual or homosexual, anal, oral, or genital contact.
    B. Sexually transmitted diseases are at epidemic levels in the United States.
    C. The nurse's first responsibility in STD control is to educate patients who may develop or have a sexually transmitted infection.
    D. Prevention of STDs is the ideal goal, but early detection and appropriate treatment continue to be considered a realistic objective.
    E. Information regarding the following types of STDs is presented:
        1. Gonorrhea
        2. Syphilis
        3. Chlamydial infection
        4. Genital herpes
        5. Genital warts
        6. Hepatitis B

LEARNING ACTIVITY

VALUES CLARIFICATION

Answer the following questions. Move into small groups and analyze and discuss your answers.

1.   As a child, when was the first time you discussed sex? With whom?

2.   As an adolescent, when was the first time you began to notice a change in your body? Were you proud of it? Did you want to change it in any way?

3.   Did your parents talk to you outright about sex? If not, what was the underlying message?

4.   Did you make an active decision to become sexually active, or did it happen spontaneously? Has "safe sex" become an important consideration?

5.   What are your feelings about sex between elderly individuals?

6.   Describe your tolerance of homosexuality as an alternate sexual life style.

7.   Describe your tolerance of a homosexual man as your fifth grade son's teacher.

8.   You discover your 10-year-old sister and her two playmates playing "doctor" in the garage. What is your response?

In your opinion,

9.   Should a married woman, who has a satisfactory sexual relationship with her husband, masturbate with a vibrator?

10.   Do most parents give their daughters as much sexual freedom as they do their sons? Should they?

11.   Do parents who give contraceptives to their adolescents present a message that having sex is okay?

12.   Are individuals who have sex change operations freaks?

13.   Does pornography lead to sexual crimes?

14.   Are oral and anal sex deviant behaviors?

15.   Do you ever have the right to refuse treatment to an AIDS patient?

PARAPHILIAS

Exhibitionism

Fetishism

Frotteurism

Pedophilia

Sexual Masochism

Sexual Sadism

Voyeurism

THE HUMAN SEXUAL RESPONSE CYCLE

Phase I: Appetitive

Phase II: Excitement

Phase III: Plateau

Phase IV: Orgasm

Phase V: Resolution

TYPES OF
SEXUAL DYSFUNCTION

SEXUAL DESIRE DISORDERS
    1. Hypoactive Sexual Desire Disorder
    2. Sexual Aversion Disorder

SEXUAL AROUSAL DISORDERS
    1. Female Sexual Arousal Disorder
    2. Male Sexual Arousal Disorder

ORGASM DISORDERS
    1. Inhibited Female Orgasm (Anorgasmia)
    2. Inhibited Male Orgasm (Retarded Ejaculation)
    3. Premature Ejaculation

SEXUAL PAIN DISORDERS
    1. Dyspareunia
    2. Vaginismus

ALTERNATIVE SEXUAL LIFE STYLES

Homosexuality

Transsexuality

Bisexuality

SEXUALLY TRANSMITTED DISEASES

Gonorrhea

Syphilis

Chlamydial Infection

Genital Herpes

Genital Warts

Hepatitis B

Acquired Immunodeficiency Syndrome (AIDS)

CHAPTER 24:   ADJUSTMENT AND IMPULSE CONTROL DISORDERS

CHAPTER FOCUS

The focus of this chapter is on nursing care of the patient with adjustment and impulse control disorders. Predisposing factors and symptomatology are explored, and nursing care is presented in the context of the five steps of the nursing process. Medical treatment modalities are also discussed.

LEARNING OBJECTIVES

After reading this chapter, the student will be able to:

1.   Discuss historical aspects and epidemiological statistics related to adjustment and impulse control disorders.
2.   Describe various types of adjustment and impulse control disorders and identify symptomatology associated with each. Use this information in patient assessment.
3.   Identify predisposing factors in the development of adjustment and impulse control disorders.
4.   Formulate nursing diagnoses and goals of care for patients with adjustment and impulse control disorders.
5.   Describe appropriate nursing interventions for behaviors associated with adjustment and impulse control disorders.
6.   Evaluate nursing care of patients with adjustment and impulse control disorders.
7.   Discuss various modalities relevant to treatment of adjustment and impulse control disorders.

KEY TERMS

adjustment disorder   pathological gambling
Gamblers Anonymous   pyromania
kleptomania   trichotillomania

CHAPTER OUTLINE/LECTURE NOTES

I.   Introduction
      A. Adjustment disorders are precipitated by an identifiable psychosocial stressor, and impulse disorders are often
          modulated directly by the severity of psychosocial stressors.
      B. Behaviors may include:
          1. Impairment in an individual's usual social and occupational functioning.
          2. Compulsive acts that may be harmful to the person or others.
II.   Historical and Epidemiological Factors
      A. Historically, patients with symptoms identified by adjustment or impulse control disorders were classified as
          having personality disturbances.
      B. The original impulse control disorders date back to the 19th century and included alcoholism, firesetting,
          homicide, and kleptomania.
      C. Adjustment disorders are quite common. Some studies indicate that adjustment disorder is the most frequent
          diagnosis given.
III. Application of the Nursing Process
      A. Adjustment disorders: background assessment data
          1. An adjustment disorder is characterized by a maladaptive reaction to an identifiable psychosocial stressor
              that occurs within three to six months after onset of the stressor.
          2. Categories are distinguished by the predominant features of the maladaptive response.
              a. Adjustment disorder with anxious mood. This category denotes a maladaptive response to a
                  psychosocial stressor in which the predominant manifestation is anxiety.
              b. Adjustment disorder with depressed mood. This category (the most common) is one of predominant

mood disturbance, although less pronounced than that of major depression.

    c.   Adjustment disorder with disturbance of conduct. Characterized by conduct in which there is violation of the rights of others or of major age-appropriate societal norms and rules.

    d.   Adjustment disorder with mixed disturbance of emotions and conduct. Predominant features of this category include mood disturbances and emotional disturbances, as well as conduct in which there is violation of the rights of others or of major age-appropriate societal norms and rules.

    e.   Adjustment disorder with mixed emotional features. Designates a subtype of adjustment disorder that is characterized by a combination of depression and anxiety or other emotions.

    f.   Adjustment disorder with physical complaints. Identifies patients who respond to major life stressors with repression and external expression of somatic symptoms.

    g.   Adjustment disorder with withdrawal. The predominant manifestation of this category is social withdrawal without significantly depressed or anxious mood.

    h.   Adjustment disorder with work (or academic) inhibition. Identifies the individual who prior to experiencing a major psychosocial stressor had been capable of performing adequately in either an occupational or academic role.

3. Predisposing factors to adjustment disorders

    a.   Biologic theory. The presence of chronic disorders, such as organic mental disorder or mental retardation, is thought to limit the general adaptive capacity of an individual.

    b.   Psychosocial theories.

        (1) Some proponents of psychoanalytic theory view adjustment disorder as a maladaptive response to stress that is caused by early childhood trauma, increased dependency, and retarded ego development.

        (2) Other psychosocial theories describe a predisposition to adjustment disorder as an inability to complete the grieving process in response to a painful life change, due to a type of "psychic overload."

    c.   Transactional model of stress adaptation. The way in which certain individuals respond to various types of stressors depends upon the type of stressor, the situational context in which the stressor occurs, and intrapersonal factors. The transactional model takes into consideration the interaction between the individual and his or her internal and external environment.

4. Nursing diagnosis, planning/implementation

    a.   Nursing intervention for the patient with adjustment disorder is aimed at assisting the individual to progress toward resolution of grief that has been generated in response to real or perceived losses.

    b.   If the adjustment disorder is in response to a change in health status, the nurse assists the patient to accept the change and make required life style modifications in order to function as independently as possible.

5. Evaluation is based on accomplishment of previously established outcome criteria.

B. Impulse control disorders: background assessment data

1. The essential features of impulse control disorders include:

    a.   Failure to resist an impulse, drive, or temptation to perform some act that is harmful to the person or others.

    b.   An increasing sense of tension or arousal before committing the act.

    c.   An experience of either pleasure, gratification, or release at the time of committing the act.

2. Five categories of impulse control disorders are described:

    a.   Intermittent explosive disorder. Characterized by a loss of control of a violent or aggressive impulse that culminates in serious assaultive acts or destruction of property.

        (1) Predisposing factors to intermittent explosive disorder include:

            (a) Biologic influences. Genetically, the disorder is more common in first degree biologic relatives of people with the disorder than in the general population. Physiologically, any central nervous system insult may predispose to the general clinical syndrome.

            (b) Psychosocial influences. Individuals with intermittent explosive disorder often have very strong identification with assaultive parental figures.

    b.   Kleptomania. Characterized by recurrent failure to resist impulses to steal objects not needed for personal use or their monetary value.

        (1) Predisposing factors to kleptomania.

            (a) Biologic influences. Brain disease and mental retardation are known on occasion to be associated with profitless stealing.

            (b) Psychosocial influences. Some kleptomaniacs report childhood memories of abandonment

(real or imagined) and a sense of lovelessness and deprivation.
- c. Pathological gambling. A chronic and progressive failure to resist impulses to gamble, and gambling behavior that compromises, disrupts, or damages personal, family, or vocational pursuits.
  - (1) Predisposing factors to pathological gambling.
    - (a) Biologic influences. Genetically, the fathers of males with the disorder and the mothers of females with the disorder are more likely to have the disorder than is the population at large. Physiologically, various neurophysiologic dysfunctions have been associated with pathological gambling.
    - (b) Psychosocial influences. Possible contributors include: inappropriate parental discipline; exposure to gambling activities as an adolescent; a high family value placed on material and financial symbols; and a lack of family emphasis on saving, planning, and budgeting. Some psychodynamicists view the pathological gambler as continuing to struggle with the oedipal complex.
- d. Pyromania. The inability to resist the impulse to set fires.
  - (1) Predisposing factors to pyromania.
    - (a) Biologic influences. Physiologic factors that may contribute include mental retardation, dementia, epilepsy, minimal brain dysfunction, and learning disabilities.
    - (b) Psychosocial influences. Psychoanalytic issues associated with impulsive firesetting include an association between firesetting and sexual gratification; concerns about inferiority, impotence, and annihilation; and unconscious anger toward a parent figure.
- e. Trichotillomania. The recurrent failure to resist impulses to pull out one's own hair.
  - (1) Predisposing factors to trichotillomania.
    - (a) Biologic influences. A family history of the disorder has been demonstrated.
    - (b) Psychosocial influences. Factors that have been considered include disturbances in mother-child relationships, fear of abandonment, and recent object loss. Another view associates the disorder with early emotional deprivation.
3. Transactional model of stress-adaptation. The etiology of impulse control disorders is most likely influenced by multiple factors.
4. Nursing diagnosis, planning/implementation.
   - a. Nursing intervention for the patient with impulse control disorder is aimed at protection of the patient and others from harm associated with aggressive impulses and assaultive behavior.
   - b. The nurse also assists the patient to learn to delay gratification and to develop more adaptive strategies for coping with stress.
5. Evaluation is based on accomplishment of previously established outcome criteria.

IV. Treatment Modalities
   A. Adjustment disorder
      1. The major goals of therapy include:
         - a. Relieving symptoms.
         - b. Achieving a level of adaptation that at least equals the level of functioning before the stressful event.
         - c. Undergoing positive change whenever possible.
      2. Types of therapy
         - a. Individual psychotherapy
         - b. Family therapy
         - c. Behavior therapy
         - d. Self-help groups
         - e. Psychopharmacology
   B. Impulse control disorders
      1. Intermittent explosive disorder
         - a. Group/family therapy
         - b. Psychopharmacology
      2. Kleptomania
         - a. Insight-oriented psychodynamic psychotherapy
         - b. Behavior therapy
      3. Pathological gambling
         - a. Behavior therapy
         - b. Psychopharmacology
         - c. Gamblers Anonymous

LEARNING ACTIVITY

CASE STUDY

Read the following case study and answer the questions that follow.

Nancy is 30 years old. She has never been married. She is a top salesperson in a major pharmaceutical company. She has an active social life, with many friends. She has had serious relationships with several men in the past, but has no significant relationship at this time. Three months ago, in a routine physical exam, the physician discovered a lump in Nancy's right breast. It was biopsied and found to be malignant. Because of the location, size, and likely metastasis to adjacent lymph nodes, Nancy chose, with the recommendation of her physician, to have a modified radical mastectomy. Since the surgery, her physical condition has progressed unremarkably. However, her mental condition has deteriorated progressively. She is sad, tired, and has trouble sleeping and concentrating. She has been unable to return to her job. She is referred to a psychiatrist, and admitted to the hospital with a diagnosis of Adjustment Disorder with Depressed Mood. She tells the nurse, "No man will ever want to have anything to do with me because of the way I look. My personal life is over."

1. Identify relevant assessment data from the information given.

2. What are the two priority nursing diagnoses for Nancy?

3. Describe some nursing interventions for assisting Nancy with the two nursing diagnoses identified.

4. Describe relevant outcome criteria for evaluating nursing care for Nancy.

TYPES OF ADJUSTMENT DISORDERS

Adjustment Disorder with Anxious Mood

Adjustment Disorder with Depressed Mood

Adjustment Disorder with Disturbance of Conduct

Adjustment Disorder with Mixed Disturbance of Emotions and Conduct

Adjustment Disorder with Mixed Emotional Features

Adjustment Disorder with Physical Complaints

Adjustment Disorder with Withdrawal

Adjustment Disorder with Work (or Academic) Inhibition

NURSING DIAGNOSES FOR PATIENTS WITH ADJUSTMENT DISORDERS

Dysfunctional Grieving

Impaired Adjustment

TYPES OF IMPULSE CONTROL DISORDERS

Intermittent Explosive Disorder

Kleptomania

Pathological Gambling

Pyromania

Trichotillomania

NURSING DIAGNOSES FOR PATIENTS WITH IMPULSE CONTROL DISORDERS

High Risk For Violence

Ineffective Individual Coping

CHAPTER 25: PSYCHOLOGICAL FACTORS AFFECTING PHYSICAL CONDITION

CHAPTER FOCUS

The focus of this chapter is on nursing care of the patient with physical conditions, the initiation or exacerbation of which are associated with psychological factors. Predisposing factors and symptomatology are explored, and nursing care is presented in the context of the five steps of the nursing process. Medical treatment modalities are also discussed.

LEARNING OBJECTIVES

After reading this chapter, the student will be able to:

1. Differentiate between somatoform and psychophysiologic disorders.
2. Identify various types of psychophysiologic disorders.
3. Discuss historic and epidemiologic statistics related to various psychophysiologic disorders.
4. Describe symptomatology associated with various psychophysiologic disorders and use this data in patient assessment.
5. Identify various predisposing factors to psychophysiologic disorders.
6. Formulate nursing diagnoses and goals of care for patients with various psychophysiologic disorders.
7. Describe appropriate nursing interventions for behaviors associated with various psychophysiologic disorders.
8. Evaluate nursing care of patients with psychophysiologic disorders.
9. Discuss various modalities relevant to treatment of psychophysiologic disorders.

KEY TERMS

autoimmune	psychophysiologic
cachexia	psychosomatic
carcinogens	type A personality
essential hypertension	type B personality
migraine personality	type C personality

CHAPTER OUTLINE/LECTURE NOTES

I. Introduction
  A. In pathophysiologic responses, evidence exists of either demonstrable organic pathology or a known pathophysiologic process. No such organic involvement can be identified in somatoform disorders.
  B. Virtually any organic disorder can be considered psychophysiologic in nature.
II. Historical Aspects
  A. Historically, mind and body have been viewed as two distinct entities, each subject to different laws of causality.
  B. Medical research shows that a change is occurring. Research associated with biological functioning is being expanded to include the psychological and social determinants of health and disease.
III. Application of the Nursing Process
  A. Types of psychophysiologic disorders: background assessment data
    1. Asthma
      a. A syndrome of airflow limitation characterized by increased responsiveness of the tracheobronchial tree to various stimuli and manifested by airway smooth muscle contraction, hypersecretion of mucous, and inflammation.
      b. Affects approximately 7 million adults and children in the U.S.

c. Predisposing factors
  (1) Biologic influences
    (a) Hereditary factors
    (b) Allergies
  (2) Psychosocial influences
    (a) Personality profile: unresolved dependence on the mother.
2. Cancer
  a. A malignant neoplasm in which the basic structure and activity of the cells have become deranged, usually due to changes in the DNA.
  b. Cancer is second leading cause of death in the U.S. today.
  c. Seven warning signs of cancer:
    (1) A change in bowel or bladder habits
    (2) A sore that does not heal
    (3) Unusual bleeding or discharge
    (4) A thickening or lump in the breast or elsewhere
    (5) Indigestion or difficulty in swallowing
    (6) An obvious change in a wart or mole
    (7) A nagging cough or hoarseness
  d. Predisposing factors
    (1) Biologic influences
      (a) Familial pattern: possible hereditary link
      (b) Continuous irritation
      (c) Exposure to carcinogens
      (d) Viruses
    (2) Psychosocial influences
      (a) Type C personality
      (b) Lack of close relationship with one or both parents
      (c) Lack of opportunity for self-gratification
3. Coronary heart disease
  a. Myocardial impairment due to an imbalance between coronary blood flow and myocardial oxygen requirements caused by changes in the coronary circulation. It is the leading cause of death in the U.S.
  b. Predisposing factors
    (1) Biologic influences
      (a) Hereditary factors
      (b) High serum lipoproteins
      (c) Life style habits: cigarette smoking, obesity, sedentary life style
    (2) Psychosocial influences
      (a) Type A personality
4. Peptic ulcer
  a. An erosion of the mucosal wall in the esophagus, stomach, duodenum, or jejunum.
  b. One in every 10 men and one in every 40 women might expect to experience signs and symptoms of peptic ulcer disease during their lifetime.
  c. The characteristic clinical manifestation is pain that is usually experienced in the upper abdomen near the midline, and may radiate to the back, sternum, or lower abdomen.
  d. Predisposing factors
    (1) Biologic influences
      (a) Hereditary factor
      (b) Environmental factors: cigarette smoking, aspirin, alcohol, steroids, and non-steroidal anti-inflammatory drugs.
    (2) Psychosocial influences
      (a) Unfulfilled dependency needs
5. Essential hypertension
  a. The persistent elevation of blood pressure for which there is no apparent cause or associated underlying disease.
  b. It is the major cause of cerebrovascular accident, cardiac disease, and renal failure.
  c. Thirty-eight percent of the population have a blood pressure of 140/90 mm Hg or higher.

d. Predisposing factors
    (1) Biologic influences
        (a) Hereditary factors
        (b) Possible imbalance of circulating vasoconstrictors and vasodilators
        (c) Increased sympathetic nervous system activity resulting in increased vasoconstriction
        (d) Impairment in sodium and water excretion
    (2) Psychosocial influences
        (a) Repressed anger

6. Migraine headache
   a. A vascular event in which pain arises from the scalp, its blood vessels, and muscles; from the dura mater and its venous sinuses; and from the blood vessels at the base of the brain.
   b. Approximately 5% of the population suffers from migraine headaches.
   c. Predisposing factors
    (1) Biologic influences
        (a) Hereditary factors
        (b) Periods of hormonal change
        (c) Certain foods, beverages, and drugs
        (d) Physical exertion
        (e) Other factors: cigarette smoking, bright lights, weather changes, high elevations, oral contraceptives, altered sleep patterns, and skipping meals
    (2) Psychosocial influences
        (a) Migraine personality

7. Obesity
   a. A body mass index (weight/height^2) that is greater than 20% above the ideal value
   b. It is estimated that approximately one out of five persons over the age of 19 years is obese
   c. Predisposing factors
    (1) Biologic influences
        (a) Hereditary factors
        (b) Lesions in the appetite and satiety centers in the hypothalamus
        (c) Hypothyroidism
        (d) Sedentary life style
    (2) Psychosocial influences
        (a) Unresolved dependency needs and fixation in the oral stage of psychosexual development.

8. Rheumatoid arthritis
   a. A chronic systemic disease characterized by inflammation of the connective tissues throughout the body.
   b. Rheumatoid arthritis affects 0.5 to 1 percent of the population in the U.S. between the ages of 20 and 80 years.
   c. Predisposing factors
    (1) Biologic influences
        (a) Hereditary factors
        (b) Possible dysfunctional immune mechanism
    (2) Psychosocial influences
        (a) Suppression of anger and hostility

9. Ulcerative Colitis
   a. A chronic mucosal inflammatory disease of the colon and rectum
   b. Incidence of the disease is approximately 5 to 7 per 100,000 population
   c. Predisposing factors
    (1) Biologic influences
        (a) Hereditary factors
        (b) Possible dysfunctional immune mechanism
    (2) Psychosocial influences
        (a) Obsessive-compulsive personality
        (b) Suppression of anger and hostility

B. Transactional model of stress adaptation
  1. The etiology of psychophysiologic disorders is most likely influenced by multiple factors.
C. Nursing diagnosis, planning/implementation

1. Nursing intervention for the patient with psychophysiologic disorders is determined by the type of disorder with which the patient presents.
2. Some nursing diagnoses common to the general category include:
   a. Ineffective individual coping
   b. Knowledge deficit
   c. Self-esteem disturbance
   d. Altered role performance
   D. Evaluation is based on accomplishment of previously established outcome criteria.
IV. Treatment Modalities
   A. Asthma
      1. Chemotherapy
      2. Individual psychotherapy
   B. Cancer
      1. Surgery
      2. Radiation therapy
      3. Chemotherapy
      4. Autogenic relaxation and mental imagery
      5. Individual psychotherapy
   C. Coronary heart disease
      1. Surgery
      2. Angioplasty
      3. Chemotherapy
      4. Behavior modification
   D. Peptic ulcer
      1. Chemotherapy
      2. Dietary intervention
      3. Surgery
      4. Individual psychotherapy
   E. Hypertension
      1. Life style changes
      2. Chemotherapy
      3. Relaxation therapy
      F. Migraine headaches
         1. Chemotherapy
         2. Relaxation therapy
         3. Dietary restrictions
         4. Behavior modification
         5. Individual psychotherapy
   G. Obesity
      1. Behavior therapy
      2. Self-help groups
      3. Pharmacological treatment
      4. Surgery
      5. Individual psychotherapy
   H. Rheumatoid arthritis
      1. Pharmacologic treatment
      2. Surgical treatment
      3. Psychological treatment
   I. Ulcerative colitis
      1. Nutritional therapy
      2. Pharmacologic treatment
      3. Surgical treatment
      4. Psychological support
V. Summary
VI. Review Questions

LEARNING ACTIVITY

Please select the most appropriate answer for each of the following questions.

1. Which of the following psychosocial influences has been correlated with the predisposition to asthma?
   a. unresolved oedipus complex
   b. underdeveloped ego
   c. punitive superego
   d. unresolved dependence on the mother

2. Type C personality characteristics include all of the following *except*:
   a. exhibits a calm, placid exterior
   b. puts others' needs before their own
   c. has a strong competitive drive
   d. holds resentment toward others for perceived "wrongs"

3. Friedman and Rosenman identified two major character traits common to individuals with Type A personality. They are:
   a. excessive competitive drive and chronic sense of time urgency
   b. unmet dependency needs and low self-esteem
   c. chronic depression and tendency toward self-pity
   d. self-sacrificing and perfectionistic

4. Which of the following statements is true about Type B personality?
   a. Their personalities are the exact opposite of Type A's.
   b. They lack the need for competition and comparison as do Type A's.
   c. They are usually less successful than Type A's.
   d. They do not perform as well under pressure as Type A's.

5. Which of the following has *not* been implicated in the etiology of peptic ulcer disease?
   a. genetics
   b. cigarette smoking
   c. allergies
   d. unfulfilled dependency needs

6. The individual with essential hypertension is thought to
   a. suppress anger and hostility.
   b. fear social interactions with others.
   c. project feelings onto the environment.
   d. deny responsibility for own behavior.

7. The "migraine personality" includes which of the following sets of characteristics?
   a. compulsive, perfectionistic, and somewhat inflexible
   b. excessively ambitious, easily aroused hostility, and highly competitive
   c. highly extroverted, impulsive, and expresses anger inappropriately
   d. chronic feelings of depression and despair, and has a tendency toward self-pity

8. The obese person is thought to be fixed in what stage of psychosexual development?
   a. oral
   b. anal
   c. phallic
   d. latency

9. The individual with ulcerative colitis has been found to have which of the following types of personality characteristics?
   a. passive-aggressive

b. obsessive-compulsive
c. antisocial-suspicious
d. hostile-aggressive

10. Individuals with ulcerative colitis and rheumatoid arthritis share which of the following personality characteristics?
a. highly negativistic
b. strongly independent
c. excessively introverted
d. unable to express anger directly

PSYCHOPHYSIOLOGIC DISORDERS

Asthma

Cancer

Coronary Heart Disease

Peptic Ulcer

Essential Hypertension

Migraine Headache

Obesity

Rheumatoid Arthritis

Ulcerative Colitis

NURSING DIAGNOSES COMMON TO PSYCHOPHYSIOLOGIC DISORDERS

Ineffective Individual Coping

Knowledge Deficit

Self-Esteem Disturbance

Altered Role Performance

CHAPTER 26:   PERSONALITY DISORDERS

CHAPTER FOCUS

The focus of this chapter is on nursing care of the patient with personality disorders. Predisposing factors and symptomatology are explored, and nursing care is presented in the context of the five steps of the nursing process. Medical treatment modalities are also discussed.

LEARNING OBJECTIVES

After reading this chapter, the student will be able to:

1.   Define *personality*.
2.   Compare stages of personality development according to Sullivan, Erikson, and Mahler.
3.   Identify various types of personality disorders.
4.   Discuss historical and epidemiological statistics related to various personality disorders.
5.   Describe symptomatology associated with borderline personality disorder and antisocial personality disorder, and use this data in patient assessment.
6.   Identify predisposing factors to borderline personality disorder and antisocial personality disorder.
8.   Describe appropriate nursing interventions for behaviors associated with borderline personality disorder and antisocial personality disorder.
9.   Evaluate nursing care of patients with borderline personality disorder and antisocial personality disorder.
10.   Discuss various modalities relevant to treatment of personality disorders.

KEY TERMS

histrionic	personality
narcissism	schizoid
object constancy	schizotypal
passive-aggressive	splitting

CHAPTER OUTLINE/LECTURE NOTES

I.   Introduction
   A.   Personality is a complex pattern of deeply embedded psychological characteristics that are largely unconscious, cannot be eradicated easily, and express themselves automatically in almost every facet of functioning.
   B.   Personality traits are enduring patterns of perceiving, relating to, and thinking about the environment and oneself, and are exhibited in a wide range of important social and personal contexts.
   C.   Personality disorders occur when these traits become inflexible and maladaptive and cause either significant functional impairment or subjective distress.

II.   Historical Aspects
   A.   The first recognition that personality disorders, apart from psychosis, were cause for their own special concern was in 1801, with the recognition that an individual can behave irrationally even when the powers of intellect are intact.
   B.   Personality disorders have been categorized into three clusters, according to the type of behavior observed.
      1.   Cluster A: behaviors that are described as odd or eccentric.
         a.   Paranoid personality disorder
         b.   Schizoid personality disorder

        c.   Schizotypal personality disorder

    2.   Cluster B: behaviors that are described as dramatic, emotional, or erratic.

        a.   Antisocial personality disorder

        b.   Borderline personality disorder

        c.   Histrionic personality disorder

        d.   Narcissistic personality disorder

    3.   Cluster C: behaviors are described as anxious or fearful.

        a.   Avoidant personality disorder

        b.   Dependent personality disorder

        c.   Obsessive compulsive personality disorder

        d.   Passive-aggressive personality disorder

III.   Application of the Nursing Process

    A.   Types of personality disorders: background assessment data

      1.   Paranoid personality disorder

        a.   A pervasive and unwarranted tendency, beginning by early adulthood and present in a variety of contexts, to interpret the actions of people as deliberately demeaning or threatening.

        b.   Such persons are constantly on guard, hypervigilant, and ready for any real or imagined threat. They trust no one, and are constantly testing the honesty of others.

        c.   Predisposing factors

           (1)   Possible genetic link.

           (2)   Subject to early parental antagonism and aggression.

      2.   Schizoid personality disorder

        a.   Characterized primarily by a profound defect in the ability to form personal relationships or to respond to others in any meaningful, emotional way.

        b.   They are indifferent to others, aloof, detached, and unresponsive to praise, criticism, or any other feelings expressed by others.

        c.   Predisposing factors

           (1)   Possible hereditary factor.

           (2)   Childhood has been characterized as bleak, cold, unempathetic, and notably lacking in nurturing.

      3.   Schizotypal personality disorder

        a.   A graver form of the pathologically less severe schizoid personality pattern.

        b.   Schizotypals are aloof and isolated and behave in a bland and apathetic manner since they experience few pleasures and have need to avoid few discomforts.

        c.   Predisposing factors

           (1)   Possible hereditary factor.

           (2)   Possible physiological influence, such as anatomic deficits or neurochemical dysfunctions within certain areas of the brain.

           (3)   Early family dynamics characterized by indifference, impassivity, or formality, leading to a pattern of discomfort with personal affection and closeness.

      4.   Antisocial personality disorder

        a.   A pattern of socially irresponsible, exploitative, and guiltless behavior, evident in the tendency to fail to conform to the law, to sustain consistent employment, to exploit and manipulate others for personal gain, to deceive, and to fail to develop stable relationships.

        b.   Predisposing factors presented later in this outline.

      5.   Borderline personality disorder

        a.   Characterized by a pattern of intense and chaotic relationships, with affective instability, fluctuating and extreme attitudes regarding other people, impulsivity, directly and indirectly self-destructive behavior, and lack of a clear or certain sense of identity, life plan, or values.

        b.   Predisposing factors presented later in this outline.

      6.   Histrionic personality disorder

        a.   Characterized by colorful, dramatic, and extroverted behavior in excitable, emotional persons.

        b.   They are self-dramatizing, attention seeking, overly gregarious, seductive, manipulative, exhibitionistic, shallow, frivolous, labile, vain, and demanding.

        c.   Predisposing factors

           (1)   Possible ease of sympathetic arousal, adrenal hyperreactivity, and neurochemical imbalances.

        (2)   Possible hereditary factor.

        (3)   Learned behavior patterns.

7.   Narcissistic personality disorder

    a.   Characterized by an exaggerated sense of self-worth.

    b.   They are overly self-centered and exploit others in an effort to fulfill their own desires.

    c.   Predisposing factors

        (1)   Family dynamics may have fostered feelings of omnipotence and grandiosity through total indulgence of the child.

8.   Avoidant personality disorder

    a.   Characterized by extreme sensitivity to rejection and social withdrawal.

    b.   They are awkward and uncomfortable in social situations. They desire to have close relationships, but cannot help believing that such will result in pain and disillusionment.

    c.   Predisposing factors

        (1)   Possible hereditary factor.

        (2)   Parental rejection and deprecation.

        (3)   Possession of a disfiguring physical illness.

9.   Dependent personality disorder

    a.   A pattern of relying excessively on others for emotional support, advice, and reassurance.

    b.   They have a notable lack of self-confidence that is often apparent in their posture, voice, and mannerisms. They are typically passive and acquiescent to the desires of others.

    c.   Predisposing factors

        (1)   Possible hereditary influence.

        (2)   Stimulation and nurturance is experienced exclusively from one source, and a singular attachment is made by the infant to the exclusion of all others.

10.   Obsessive compulsive personality disorder

    a.   Characterized by inflexibility about the way in which things must be done, and a devotion to productivity at the exclusion of personal pleasure

    b.   They are especially concerned with matters of organization and efficiency, and tend to be rigid and unbending about rules and procedures.

    c.   Predisposing factors

        (1)   Overcontrol by parents, with notable lack of positive reinforcement for acceptable behavior and frequent punishment for undesirable behavior.

11.   Passive aggressive personality disorder

    a.   A pervasive pattern of passive resistance, expressed indirectly rather than directly, to demands for adequate social and occupational performance.

    b.   They are passively resistant to authority, demands, obligations, and responsibilities by such behaviors as dawdling, procrastination, and "forgetting."

    c.   Predisposing factors

        (1)   Contradictory parental attitudes and inconsistent training methods.

IV.   Borderline Personality Disorder

    A.   Designated as "borderline" because of the tendency of these patients to fall on the border between neuroses and psychoses.

    B.   They are most strikingly identified by the intensity and instability of their affect and behavior.

    C.   Common behaviors include:

        1.   Chronic depression

        2.   Inability to be alone

        3.   Clinging and distancing behaviors

        4.   Splitting

        5.   Manipulation

        6.   Self-destructive behaviors

        7.   Impulsivity

    D.   Predisposing factors

        1.   According to Margaret Mahler's Theory of Object Relations, the individual with borderline personality disorder becomes fixed in the rapprochement phase of development (16 to 24 months). The child fails to achieve the task of autonomy.

    E.   Nursing diagnosis, planning/implementation

        1.   Nursing intervention for the patient with borderline personality disorder is aimed at protection of the

patient from self-mutilation.
2. The nurse also seeks to assist the patient advance in the development of personality by confronting his or her true source of internalized anger.
F. Evaluation is based on accomplishment of previously established outcome criteria.

V. Antisocial Personality Disorder
A. Sometimes called sociopathic or psychopathic behavior.
B. Usually only seen in clinical settings when they are admitted by court order for psychological evaluation.
C. Most frequently encountered in prisons, jails, and rehabilitation services.
D. Common behaviors include:
1. Exploitation and manipulation of others for personal gain
2. Belligerent and argumentative
3. Lacks remorse
4. Unable to delay gratification
5. Low tolerance for frustration
6. Inconsistent work or academic performance
7. Failure to conform to societal norms
8. Impulsive and reckless
9. Inability to function as a responsible parent
10. Inability to form lasting monogamous relationship
E. Predisposing factors
1. Possible biogenic influence
2. Having a sociopathic or alcoholic father
3. Behavior disordered as a child
4. Parental deprivation during the first 5 years of life
5. Inconsistent parenting
6. History of severe physical abuse
7. Extreme poverty
F. Nursing diagnosis, planning/implementation
1. Nursing intervention for the patient with antisocial personality disorder is aimed at protection of others from the patient's aggression and hostility.
2. The nurse also seeks to assist the patient to delay gratification by setting limits on unacceptable behavior.
G. Evaluation is based on accomplishment of previously established outcome criteria.

VI. Treatment Modalities for Patients with Personality Disorders
A. Interpersonal psychotherapy
B. Psychoanalytic psychotherapy
C. Milieu or group therapy
D. Behavior therapy
E. Psychopharmacology

VII. Summary
VIII. Review Questions

LEARNING ACTIVITY

Match the personality disorder most commonly associated with the behaviors described on the right.

_____ 1. Paranoid personality disorder

_____ 2. Schizoid personality disorder

_____ 3. Schizotypal personality disorder

_____ 4. Antisocial personality disorder

_____ 5. Borderline personality disorder

_____ 6. Histrionic personality disorder

_____ 7. Narcissistic personality disorder

_____ 8. Avoidant personality disorder

_____ 9. Dependent personality disorder

_____ 10. Obsessive compulsive personality disorder

_____ 11. Passive aggressive personality disorder

a. Shows no remorse for exploitation and manipulation of others

b. Accepts a job he does not want to do, then does a poor job and delays past the deadline

c. Believes she is entitled to special privileges others do not deserve

d. They are suspicious of all others with whom they come in contact

e. Swallows a bottle of pills after therapist leaves on vacation

f. Believes he has a "sixth sense," and can know what others are thinking

g. Allows others to make all her important decisions for her

h. Refuses to enter into a relationship due to fear of rejection

i. Demonstrates highly emotional and overly dramatic behaviors

j. Has a lifelong pattern of social withdrawal

k. Believes everyone must follow the rules and that the rules can be "bent" for no one . . . ever

PERSONALITY DISORDERS

CLUSTER A (ODD OR ECCENTRIC BEHAVIOR)
    a.   Paranoid Personality Disorder
    b.   Schizoid Personality Disorder
    c.   Schizotypal Personality Disorder

CLUSTER B (DRAMATIC, EMOTIONAL OR ERRATIC BEHAVIOR)
    a.   Antisocial Personality Disorder
    b.   Borderline Personality Disorder
    c.   Histrionic Personality Disorder
    d.   Narcissistic Personality Disorder

CLUSTER C (ANXIOUS OR FEARFUL BEHAVIOR)
    a.   Avoidant Personality Disorder
    b.   Dependent Personality Disorder
    c.   Obsessive Compulsive Personality Disorder
    d.   Passive Aggressive Personality Disorder

NURSING DIAGNOSES FOR PATIENTS WITH BORDERLINE PERSONALITY DISORDER

High Risk for Self-Mutilation

Dysfunctional Grieving

Impaired Social Interaction

Personality Identity Disturbance

Anxiety (Severe to Panic)

Self-Esteem Disturbance

NURSING DIAGNOSES FOR PATIENTS WITH ANTISOCIAL PERSONALITY DISORDER

High Risk for Violence: Directed at Others

Defensive Coping

Self-Esteem Disturbance

Impaired Social Interaction

Knowledge Deficit

CHAPTER 27:   THE AGING INDIVIDUAL

CHAPTER FOCUS

The focus of this chapter is on nursing care of the aging individual. Various theories of aging and symptomatology associated with the normal aging process are presented. Special concerns of the elderly are discussed. Nursing care is described in the context of the five steps of the nursing process.

LEARNING OBJECTIVES

After reading this chapter, the student will be able to:

1. Discuss societal perspectives on aging.
2. Describe an epidemiologic profile of aging in the United States.
3. Discuss various theories of aging.
4. Describe aspects of the normal aging process:
    a. biologic
    b. psychologic
    c. sociocultural
    d. sexual
5. Discuss retirement as a special concern to the aging individual.
6. Explain personal and sociological perspectives of long-term care of the aging individual.
7. Describe the problem of elder abuse as it exists in today's society.
8. Discuss the implications of the increasing number of suicides among the elderly population.
9. Apply the steps of the nursing process to the care of aging individuals.

KEY TERMS

attachment	"granny-dumping"
bereavement overload	long-term memory
disengagement	Medicaid
geriatrics	Medicare
gerontology	menopause
geropsychiatry	osteoporosis
"granny-bashing"	short-term memory

CHAPTER OUTLINE/LECTURE NOTES

I.   Introduction
      A.   Growing old is not popular in the youth-oriented American culture.
      B.   Sixty-six million "baby boomers" will reach their 65th birthdays by the year 2030, placing more emphasis on the needs of an aging population.
II.   How Old is Old?
      A.   Our prehistoric ancestors probably had a life span of 40 years, with average life span around 18 years.
      B.   By 1985, the average life expectancy at birth was 71.2 years for men and 78.2 years for women.
      C.   Myths and stereotypes affect the way in which elderly people are treated in our culture.
      D.   Whether one is considered "old" must be self-determined, based on variables such as attitude, mental health, physical health, and degree of independence.
III. Epidemiologic Statistics
      A.   Population

1. In 1990, Americans 65 years of age or older numbered 31.2 million, representing 12.6% of the population.
2. By 2030, this number is projected at about 66 million, or 21.8 percent of the population.
   B. Marital status
   1. In 1990, 77 percent of men and 42 percent of women 65 or over were married.
   2. There were five times as many widows as widowers.
   C. Living arrangements
   1. The majority of individuals age 65 or over live alone, with spouse, or with relatives.
   D. Economic status
   1. About 3.7 million persons age 65 or over were below the poverty level in 1990.
   E. Employment
   1. Individuals age 65 or over constituted 2.8 percent of the U.S. labor force in 1990.
   F. Health status
   1. The number of days in which usual activities are restricted because of illness or injury increases with age.
   2. Emotional and mental illnesses also increase over the life cycle.
IV. Theories of Aging
   A. Biologic theories
   1. The exhaustion theory
   2. The accumulation theory
   3. The biologic programming theory
   4. The error theory
   5. The cross-linkage or eversion theory
   6. The immunologic theory
   7. The "aging clock" theory
   8. The free radical theory
   B. Psychosocial theories
   1. The activity theory of aging
   2. Continuity theory
   3. Personality theories
V. The Normal Aging Process (Knowledge Base/Background Assessment Data)
   A. Biologic aspects of aging. Changes are observed in:
   1. Skin
   2. Cardiovascular system
   3. Respiratory system
   4. Musculoskeletal system
   5. Gastrointestinal system
   6. Endocrine system
   7. Genitourinary system
   8. Immune system
   9. Nervous system
   10. Sensory systems
   B. Psychologic aspects of aging
   1. Memory functioning
   2. Intellectual functioning
   3. Learning ability
   4. Adaptation to the tasks of aging
   C. Sociocultural aspects of aging
   1. The elderly in virtually all cultures share some basic needs and interests:
      a. To live as long as possible or at least until life's satisfactions no longer compensate for its privations.
      b. To get some release from the necessity of wearisome exertion at hum-drum tasks and to have protection from too great exposure to physical hazards.
      c. To safeguard or even strengthen any prerogatives acquired in mid-life, such as skills, possessions, rights, authority, and prestige.
      d. To remain active participants in the affairs of life in either operational or supervisory roles, any sharing in group interests being preferred to idleness and indifference.

    e. To withdraw from life when necessity requires it, as timely, honorably, and comfortably as possible.

    2. In some cultures, the aged are the most powerful, the most engaged, and the most respected members of the society. This has not been the case in the American culture.

  D. Sexual aspects of aging

    1. Americans have grown up in a society that has liberated sexual expression for all other age groups, but still retains certain Victorian standards regarding sexual expression by the elderly.

    2. Cultural stereotypes play a large part in the misperception many people hold regarding sexuality of the aged.

    3. Physical changes associated with sexuality

      a. Changes in the female

      b. Changes in the male

    4. Sexual behavior in the elderly

VI. Special Concerns of the Elderly

  A. Retirement

    1. Social implications

    2. Economic implications

  B. Long-term care

    1. Potential need for services are predicted by the following factors:

      a. Age. The 65+ population is often viewed as one important long-term care target group.

      b. Health. The requirement for ongoing assistance from another human being is a consideration.

      c. Mental health status. Symptoms that would render the individual incapable of meeting the demands of daily living independently place him or her at risk.

      d. Socioeconomic and demographic factors. Lower socioeconomic status, being Caucasian and female are considered risk factors for long-term care.

      e. Marital status, living arrangements, and the informal support network. Living alone without resources for home care and few or no relatives living nearby to provide informal care are factors of high risk for institutionalization.

    2. Attitudinal factors

      a. Old persons in general are opposed to the use of institutions. Many view them as "places to go to die."

  C. Elder abuse

    1. It has been suggested that approximately 700,000 to 1 million elderly persons experience physical, verbal, sexual, or other kinds of abuse every year.

    2. The abuser is most often a relative who lives with the elderly person and is likely to be the assigned caregiver.

    3. Factors that contribute to abuse

      a. Longer life

      b. Dependency

      c. Stress

      d. Learned violence

    4. Identifying elder abuse

  D. Suicide

    1. Persons over 65 years of age represent a disproportionately high percentage of individuals who commit suicide.

    2. Seventeen percent of all suicides are committed by this age group, and suicide is the 10th most common cause of death in the elderly.

    3. The group at highest risk appears to be white males who are recently bereaved, living alone, in frail health, and fearful of becoming a financial burden on their relatives.

VII. Application of the Nursing Process

  A. Assessment. Assessment of the elderly must consider the possible biologic, psychologic, sociocultural, and sexual changes that occur in the normal aging process.

    1. Age alone does not preclude that these changes have occurred, and each patient must be assessed as a unique individual.

  B. Nursing diagnosis, planning/implementation

    1. Nursing care of the aging individual is aimed at protection from injury due to age-related physical changes or altered thought processes related to cerebral changes.

    2. The nurse is also concerned with preservation of dignity and self-esteem in an individual who may have

come to be dependent upon others for his or her survival.
3. Assistance is provided with self-care deficits while encouraging independence to the best of his or her ability.
C. Evaluation is based on accomplishment of previously established outcome criteria.
VIII. Summary
IX. Review Questions

LEARNING ACTIVITY

CASE STUDY

Read the following case study and answer the questions that follow.

    Seventy-seven year old Angie had been a widow for 20 years. She was fiercely independent, and had run her small farm with minimal assistance since her husband died. In the last few years, her children had noticed that Angie had become increasingly forgetful. First she began forgetting the birthdays of her children and grandchildren, which was highly unlike her. Recently, she forgot that she was supposed to visit her son and his family, and failed to show up at the designated time. Last week when her daughter visited, she found a tea kettle on the stove that had burned dry when Angie forgot she had started it. Yesterday, her daughter received a call from Angie's nearest neighbor who found Angie wandering around in his field unprotected from the cold. At Angie's children's request, the family physician admits Angie to the hospital, where she is placed on the geropsychiatric unit.

1.   Identify relevant assessment data from the information given.

2.   What are the two priority nursing diagnoses for Angie?

3.   Describe some nursing interventions for assisting Angie with the two nursing diagnoses identified.

4.   Describe relevant outcome criteria for evaluating nursing care for Angie.

BIOLOGICAL ASPECTS OF AGING

Skin

Cardiovascular System

Respiratory System

Musculoskeletal System

Gastrointestinal System

Endocrine System

Genitourinary System

Immune System

Nervous System

Sensory Systems

PSYCHOLOGICAL ASPECTS OF AGING

MEMORY FUNCTIONING

INTELLECTUAL FUNCTIONING

LEARNING ABILITY

ADAPTATION TO THE TASKS OF AGING
    a. Loss and Grief
    b. Attachment and Disengagement
    c. Maintenance of Self-Identity
    d. Dealing with Death
    e. Psychiatric Disorders in Later Life

NURSING DIAGNOSES FOR THE ELDERLY PATIENT

Potential for Trauma

Altered Thought Processes

Self-Care Deficit

Caregiver Role Strain

Self-Esteem Disturbance

Sensory-Perceptual Alteration

CHAPTER 28:   THE INDIVIDUAL WITH HIV/AIDS

CHAPTER FOCUS

The focus of this chapter is on nursing care of the individual with HIV/AIDS. Predisposing factors and symptomatology associated with the disease are explored, and nursing care is presented in the context of the five steps of the nursing process. Various treatment modalities are also discussed.

LEARNING OBJECTIVES

After reading this chapter, the student will be able to:

1. Differentiate between human immunodeficiency virus (HIV), acquired immune deficiency syndrome (AIDS), and AIDS-related complex (ARC).
2. Describe the pathophysiology incurred by the HIV.
3. Discuss historical perspectives associated with AIDS.
4. Relate epidemiological statistics associated with AIDS.
5. Identify predisposing factors to AIDS.
6. Describe symptomatology associated with HIV, AIDS, and ARC, and use this data in patient assessment.
7. Formulate nursing diagnoses and goals of care for patients with AIDS.
8. Describe appropriate nursing interventions for patients with AIDS.
9. Evaluate nursing care of patients with AIDS.
10. Discuss various modalities relevant to treatment of patients with AIDS.

KEY TERMS

acquired immune deficiency syndrome
AIDS dementia complex (ADC)
AIDS-related complex
azidothymidine (AZT)
HIV wasting syndrome
hospice
human immunodeficiency virus

Kaposi's sarcoma
opportunistic infection
persistent generalized lymphadenopathy
pneumocystic pneumonia (PCP)
seroconversion
T4-lymphocytes
universal precautions

CHAPTER OUTLINE/LECTURE NOTES

I.   Introduction
    A.   Acquired immune deficiency syndrome (AIDS) was recognized as a lethal clinical syndrome in 1981.
    B.   It has grown to epidemic proportions and is the number one health priority in the U.S. today.
    C.   The human immunodeficiency virus (HIV) is the etiological agent that produces the immunosuppression resulting in AIDS.
II.   Pathophysiology Incurred by the HIV Virus
    A.   Normal immune response
        1.   Cells responsible for nonspecific immune reactions include neutrophils, monocytes, and macrophages.
        2.   Specific immune mechanisms are divided into two major types:
            a.   The cellular response (controlled by the T-lymphocytes, or T-cells).
            b.   The humoral response (controlled by the B-lymphocytes, or B-cells)
    B.   The immune response to HIV
        1.   The HIV infects the T4 lymphocytes, thereby destroying the very cells the body needs to direct an attack on the virus.

2. Normal T4 count is 600-1200 mm³.

3. It is not uncommon for someone with advanced HIV disease to present with a T4 count below 10 mm³.

III. Historical Aspects

    A. First described in the CDC's *Mortality Weekly Report* of June 5, 1981.

    B. First identified in homosexual and bisexual men in California and New York.

    C. Soon began appearing in heterosexual IV drug users and hemophiliacs.

    D. May have origin in Africa with a virus called simian T-cell leukemia virus found in monkeys and apes.

    E. Appears now in virtually every major country in the world.

IV. Epidemiological Statistics

    A. Worldwide, 8 to 10 million adults and a million children have been infected by HIV.

    B. Projections are that by the year 2000, 50 to 100 million people could be infected unless effective measures are taken to slow the transmission.

    C. About 1 million people are infected with HIV in the U.S. and more than 160,000 cases of AIDS have been reported.

    D. It has been projected that this number will increase to 365,000 by the end of 1992.

    E. The largest number of cases are reported to be in Africa and the United States.

V. Predisposing Factors

    A. The etiologic agent associated with AIDS is the HIV.

    B. Routes of transmission include sexual, bloodborne, and perinatal transmission.

        1. Sexual transmission

            a. Heterosexual transmission

            b. Homosexual transmission

        2. Bloodbourne transmission

            a. Transfusion with blood products

            b. Transmission by needles infected with HIV

                (1) IV drug users

                (2) Accidental needle sticks by health care workers

        3. Perinatal transmission

            a. Transplacental

            b. Exposure to maternal blood and vaginal secretions during delivery.

            c. Through breast feeding

        4. Other possible modes of transmission

VI. Application of the Nursing Process

    A. Background assessment data

        1. Acute HIV infection. A characteristic syndrome of symptoms that occurs from 6 days to 6 weeks following exposure to the virus. May include fever, myalgia, malaise, lymphadenopathy, sore throat, anorexia, nausea and vomiting, headaches, photophobia, skin rash, and diarrhea.

        2. Asymptomatic infection. Following the acute infection, individuals progress to an asymptomatic stage. They remain in this stage for 10 or more years.

        3. Persistent generalized lymphadenopathy (PGL). Defined as lymph nodes greater than 1 cm in diameter at two extrainguinal sites persisting for 3 months or longer, not attributable to other causes, and not associated with other substantial constitutional symptoms. May also include fever, night sweats, weight loss, and an enlarged spleen.

        4. AIDS-related complex. No longer used as a clinical description. Used to be considered a disease of HIV-infected individuals that did not fit the CDC's classification of full-blown AIDS. Symptoms such as fever, night sweats, weight loss, fatigue, and lymphadenopathy in the absence of an opportunistic infection or Kaposi's sarcoma were known formerly as ARC.

        5. HIV wasting syndrome. Identified by the CDC as having one or more of the following with absence of concurrent illness other than HIV infection: fever and weakness for more than 30 days, weight loss of > 10% of body weight, chronic diarrhea for more than one month.

        6. Opportunistic infections. A defining characteristic of AIDS.

        7. Malignancies. Common in the immunocompromised state produced by the HIV.

            a. Kaposi's sarcoma

            b. Non-Hodgkin's lymphoma

        8. Altered mental states

            a. Delirium

            b. Depressive syndromes

        c. AIDS dementia complex (ADC)
- B. Psychosocial implication of HIV/AIDS
- C. Nursing diagnosis, planning/implementation
  1. Nursing intervention for the patient with HIV/AIDS is aimed at maximizing patient safety and comfort.
  2. The nurse is also concerned with assisting the family to deal with the newly-acquired diagnosis for their loved one.
  3. Patient and family education related to protection of the patient and others from infection is also an important aspect of nursing care.
- D. Evaluation is based on accomplishment of previously established outcome criteria.

VII. Treatment Modalities
- A. Pharmacology
  1. Antiviral therapy
  2. Azidothymidine (AZT)
  3. Other chemotherapeutic agents
- B. Universal infection precautions
- C. Hospice care
  1. Multidisciplinary team
  2. Pain and symptom management
  3. Emotional support
  4. Pastoral and spiritual care
  5. Bereavement counseling
  6. Twenty-four-hour on-call
  7. Staff support

VIII. Summary

IX. Review Questions

LEARNING ACTIVITY

ACQUIRED IMMUNE DEFICIENCY SYNDROME

Identify the following key terms associated with acquired immune deficiency syndrome with the descriptions listed below. The first one is completed as an example.

a. AIDS dementia complex
b. AIDS-related complex
c. azidothymidine (AZT)
d. human immunodeficiency virus
e. Kaposi's sarcoma
f. seroconversion
g. T4 lymphocytes

h. Acute HIV infection
i. Asymptomatic infection
j. universal precautions
k. persistent generalized lymphadenopathy (PGL)
l. hospice
m. HIV wasting syndrome

___i___ 1. Period of time following acute HIV infection in which the individual experiences no symptoms. May last 10 years or more.

_____ 2. A syndrome that includes fever, excessive weight loss, and chronic diarrhea.

_____ 3. A type of malignancy common to AIDS patients in which tumor-type lesions may form on any body surface or in the viscera.

_____ 4. The time at which antibodies to the HIV virus may be detected in the blood.

_____ 5. An organization that dedicates itself to the provision of palliative and supportive care during the final stages of illness and during bereavement.

_____ 6. The most widely used antiviral agent used in the treatment of HIV infection.

_____ 7. The controlling element of the cellular immune response, which is the major target of the HIV.

_____ 8. The etiological agent that produces the immunosuppression of acquired immune deficiency syndrome.

_____ 9. A diagnosis that is no longer used clinically, but which is used to identify cases that did not fit the criteria for AIDS according to the CDC.

_____ 10. A syndrome of painful, swollen lymph nodes in at least two extrainguinal sites, persisting for 3 months or longer.

_____ 11. Guidelines published by the CDC for prevention of HIV transmission in health care setting.

_____ 12. A syndrome of pathological changes in cognition, behavior, and motor ability that become more severe with progression of HIV disease.

_____ 13. A characteristic syndrome of symptoms that occur from 6 days to 6 weeks following exposure to the virus.

ROUTES OF HIV TRANSMISSION

1. **SEXUAL TRANSMISSION**
   a. Heterosexual Transmission
   b. Homosexual Transmission

2. **BLOODBORNE TRANSMISSION**
   a. Transfusion with Blood Products
   b. Transmission by Infected Needles
      -- IV Drug Users
      -- Accidental Needle Sticks

3. **PERINATAL TRANSMISSION**
   a. Transplacental
   b. Exposure to Maternal Secretions During Delivery
   c. Through Breast Feeding

MANIFESTATIONS OF HIV INFECTION

Acute HIV Infection

Asymptomatic Infection

Persistent Generalized Lymphadenopathy

AIDS-Related Complex

HIV Wasting Syndrome

Opportunistic Infections

Malignancies

Altered Mental States

NURSING DIAGNOSES FOR THE PATIENT WITH HIV/AIDS

Altered Protection

Altered Family Processes

Knowledge Deficit

Altered Thought Processes

High Risk for Self-Directed Violence

CHAPTER 29: VICTIMS OF VIOLENCE

CHAPTER FOCUS

The focus of this chapter is on nursing care of victims of violence. Predisposing factors and symptomatology are explored, and nursing care is presented in the context of the five steps of the nursing process. Various treatment modalities are also discussed.

LEARNING OBJECTIVES

After reading this chapter, the student will be able to:

1. Discuss historical perspectives associated with woman battering, child abuse, and sexual assault.
2. Describe epidemiological statistics associated with woman battering, child abuse, and sexual assault.
3. Discuss characteristics of victims and victimizers.
4. Identify predisposing factors to victimization.
5. Describe physical and psychological effects on the victim of woman battering, child abuse, and sexual assault.
6. Identify nursing diagnoses, goals of care, and appropriate nursing interventions for care of victims of woman battering, child abuse, and sexual assault.
7. Evaluate nursing care of victims of woman battering, child abuse, and sexual assault.
8. Discuss various modalities relevant to treatment of victims of violence.

KEY TERMS

battering	incest
child sexual abuse	marital rape
compounded rape reaction	physical neglect
controlled response pattern	rape
cycle of battering	safe house/shelter
date rape	sexual exploitation of a child
emotional injury	silent rape reaction
emotional neglect	statutory rape
expressed response pattern	

CHAPTER OUTLINE/LECTURE NOTES

I. Introduction
    A. Violence is the victimization of one person against another.
    B. Battering is the single most common cause of injury to women.
    C. An increase in the incidence of child abuse has been documented.
    D. Rape is thought to be vastly underreported.
II. Historical Perspectives
    A. Wife and child abuse arrived in the U.S. with the Puritans. Women and children were viewed as personal property of men.
    B. The notion of women as subordinate and subservient to men, as well as that of "spare the rod and spoil the child," was supported by the Bible.
    C. Not until the second half of the twentieth century has legal protection been available for victims of violence.
III. Predisposing Factors
    A. Biologic theories
        1. Neurophysiologic influences. The limbic system of the brain has been implicated as an area that, when

stimulated, produces evidence of hostility and aggression.
2. Biochemical influences. Certain neurotransmitters, including epinephrine, norepinephrine, dopamine, serotonin, and acetylcholine, have been implicated in the regulation of aggressive impulses.
3. Genetic influences. A possible hereditary factor may be involved. The genetic karyotype XYY has also been implicated.
4. Disorders of the brain. Aggressive and violent behavior has been correlated with OBS, brain tumors, brain trauma, encephalitis, and temporal lobe epilepsy.
B. Psychologic theories
1. Psychoanalytic theory. Unmet needs for satisfaction and security result in an underdeveloped ego and a poor self-concept. Aggression and violence supply the individual with a dose of power and prestige that increases self-esteem.
2. Learning theory. Children learn to behave by imitating their role models. Individuals who were abused as children or whose parents disciplined with physical punishment are more likely to behave in a violent manner as adults.
C. Sociocultural theories
1. Societal influences. Aggressive behavior is primarily a product of one's culture and social structure. The American culture was founded upon a general acceptance of violence as a means of solving problems.
2. Societal influences also contribute to violence when individuals come to realize that their needs and desires cannot be met through conventional (legal) means.
IV. Application of the Nursing Process: Background Assessment Data
A. Battered women
1. Woman battering has been defined as "severe, deliberate and repeated demonstrable physical violence inflicted on a woman by a man with whom she has or has had an intimate relationship."
2. Profile of the victim. Battered women represent all age, racial, religious, cultural, educational, and socioeconomic groups. They often have low self-esteem. They may be without adequate support systems. Many grew up in violent homes.
3. Profile of the victimizer. Men who batter are generally characterized as persons with low self-esteem, pathologically jealous, presenting a "dual personality," exhibiting limited coping ability, and severe stress reactions. The spouse is viewed as a personal possession.
4. A cycle of battering. Three distinct phases:
a. Phase I. The Tension-Building Phase
b. Phase II. The Acute Battering Incident
c. Phase III. Calm, Loving, Respite (Honeymoon) Phase
5. Why do they stay? The most frequent response to this question is that they fear for their life or the lives of their children. Other reasons given include a lack of support network for leaving, religious beliefs, and a lack of financial independence to support themselves and their children.
B. Child abuse
1. Physical injury. Any non-accidental physical injury, caused by the parent or caregiver.
a. Physical signs
b. Behavioral signs
2. Emotional injury. A pattern of behavior on the part of the parent or caretaker that results in serious impairment of the child's social, emotional, or intellectual functioning.
a. Behavioral indicators
3. Neglect
a. Physical neglect. Refers to the failure on the part of the parent or caregiver to provide for that child's basic needs, such as food, clothing, shelter, medical/dental care, and supervision.
(1) Physical/behavioral indicators
b. Emotional neglect. Refers to a chronic failure by the parent or caregiver to provide the child with the hope, love, and support necessary for the development of a sound, healthy personality.
(1) Behavioral indicators
4. Sexual abuse of a child. Defined as "sexual involvement imposed upon a child by an adult who has greater power, knowledge, and resources."
a. Sexual exploitation of a child. When a child is induced or coerced into engaging in sexually explicit conduct for the purpose of promoting any performance.
b. Sexual abuse. When a child is being used for the sexual pleasure of an adult (parent or caretaker) or any other person.

c. Incest. Sexual exploitation of a child under 18 years of age by a relative or a non-relative who holds a position of trust in the family.

   d. Indicators of sexual abuse

     (1) Physical indicators

     (2) Behavioral indicators

5. Characteristics of the abuser

   a. Parents who abuse their children were likely abused as children themselves.

   b. Retarded ego development, lack of knowledge of adequate childrearing practices, lack of empathy, and low self-esteem.

   c. Certain environmental influences, such as numerous stresses, poverty, social isolation, and an absence of adequate support systems, may predispose to child abuse.

6. The incestual relationship

   a. Often there is an impaired spousal relationship.

   b. Father is often domineering, impulsive, and physically abusing.

   c. Mother is commonly passive, submissive, and denigrates her role of wife and mother. She is often aware of, or at least suspects, the incestual relationship, but uses denial or keeps quiet out of fear of being abused by her husband.

7. The adult survivor of incest

   a. Common characteristics:

     (1) A fundamental lack of trust that arises out of an unsatisfactory mother-child relationship.

     (2) Low self-esteem and a poor sense of identity.

     (3) Absence of pleasure with sexual activity.

     (4) Promiscuity

C. Sexual assault

1. Rape is an act of aggression, not passion. It is identified by the use of force and executed "against the person's will."

   a. Date rape. Applied to sexual assault in which the rapist is known to the victim.

   b. Marital rape. Sexual violence directed at a marital partner against that person's will.

   c. Statutory rape. Unlawful intercourse between a male over age 16 and a female under the age of consent.

2. Profile of the victimizer

   a. The mother of the rapist has been described as "seductive but rejecting" toward her child. She is overbearing, with seductive undertones, but is quick to withdraw her "love" and attention when he goes against her wishes. Her dominance over her son often continues into his adult life.

   b. Many rapists report growing up in abusive homes. Even when the abuse was discharged by the father, the rapist's anger is directed toward the mother for not providing adequate protection from the father's abuse.

3. The victim

   a. Rape can occur at any age. The highest risk group appears to be between 16 and 24 years.

   b. Most victims are single women, and the attack occurs near their own neighborhood.

   c. When the attack is a "stranger rape," a victim is not chosen for any reason having to do with her appearance or her behavior, but simply because she happened to be in that place at that particular time.

   d. The presence of a weapon (real or perceived) appears to be the principal measure of the degree to which a woman resists her attacker.

   e. Victim responses:

     (1) Expressed response pattern

     (2) Controlled response pattern

     (3) Compounded reaction

     (4) Silent rape reaction

V. Nursing Diagnoses, Planning/Implementation

A. Nursing intervention for the victim of violence is to provide shelter and promote reassurance of his or her safety.

B. Other nursing concerns include:

1. Tending to physical injuries

2. Staying with the patient to provide security

3. Assisting the patient to recognize options

LEARNING ACTIVITY

VICTIMS OF VIOLENCE

Match terms on the right to the situations they describe on the left.

_____ 1. John likes to brag of his sexual conquests to his friends. When Alice rejected his sexual advances on their first date, he became angry and forced intercourse with her.

a. Physical injury

b. Compounded rape reaction

_____ 2. Alice tells no one about the encounter with John. She suppresses her anxiety and tries to pretend it didn't happen.

c. Wife battering

_____ 3. Harry is 28 years old. He is very flattered when 15-year-old Lisa pays attention to him at a party. After the party, he takes her to his home, where she agrees to have sex with him.

d. Date rape

e. Expressed response pattern

_____ 4. At 9 p.m., Jack gets home from the bar where he had gone after work with his friends. He is intoxicated, and when he finds his dinner cold, he slaps his wife across the face, knocks her down, and kicks her in the side.

f. Incest

g. Marital rape

_____ 5. Jack pulls his wife to their bed, and against her protests, forces intercourse with her, yelling, "You can't say no to me! You're my wife!"

h. Statutory rape

i. Silent rape

_____ 6. Janie is 6 years old. Her father left home a year ago and has never returned. Her mother frequently says to Janie, "See what you did? If you had been a better girl, Daddy wouldn't have left us!"

j. Emotional injury

k. Emotional neglect

_____ 7. Janie attempts to establish a relationship with her mother, but whenever Janie approaches her mother for interaction, her mother yells, "Get away from me! I don't want to have anything to do with bad little girls!"

l. Physical neglect

_____ 8. Janie has open sores on her buttocks. She tells the babysitter, "My mommy made them with her cigarette."

_____ 9. Janie comes to school in the snow without a coat. When the teacher asks her where her coat is, Janie replies, "I don't have one."

_____ 10. Scarlet is 15 years old. She is sent to the school nurse by her homeroom teacher. She is obviously having symptoms of a panic attack. Upon becoming calmer, Scarlet explains to the nurse that Frank just asked her for her first date. With much encouragement,

the nurse learns that Scarlet's father has been
coming into her bed at night for 5 years now. At
first he just touched and fondled her, but last
year he began having intercourse with her.

_____ 11. After being raped by a man in the deserted laundry
room of her apartment building, Carol is taken to
the hospital by her roommate. Carol is sobbing and
yelling, "He had no right to do that to me!" She is
tense, and is fearful of any man who comes near her.

_____ 12. Carol's physical wounds heal, but in subsequent
weeks, she becomes increasingly fearful. She is
overcome with despair and talks of taking her
life. She drinks a great deal of alcohol to help
her get through each day.

CYCLE OF BATTERING

Phase I.
The Tension-Building Phase

Phase II.
The Acute Battering Incident

Phase III.
Calm, Loving, Respite (Honeymoon) Phase

CHILD ABUSE

1. INJURY
a. Physical
b. Emotional

2. NEGLECT
a. Physical
b. Emotional

3. SEXUAL ABUSE

NURSING DIAGNOSES FOR VICTIMS OF VIOLENCE

Rape Trauma Syndrome

Powerlessness

Altered Growth and Development

CHAPTER 30: ETHICAL AND LEGAL ISSUES IN PSYCHIATRIC/ MENTAL HEALTH NURSING

CHAPTER FOCUS

The focus of this chapter is on ethical and legal issues that affect psychiatric/mental health nursing. Ethical theories, dilemmas, and principles are explored as a foundation for decision-making. Various types of law are defined, and situations for which nurses may be held liable are discussed.

LEARNING OBJECTIVES

After reading this chapter, the student will be able to:

1. Differentiate between ethics, morals, values, and rights.
2. Discuss ethical theories, including utilitarianism, Kantianism, Christian ethics, natural law theories, and ethical egoism.
3. Define *ethical dilemma.*
4. Discuss the ethical principles of autonomy, beneficence, nonmaleficence, and justice.
5. Utilize an ethical decision-making model to make an ethical decision.
6. Describe ethical issues relevant to psychiatric/mental health nursing.
7. Define *statutory law* and *common law.*
8. Differentiate between civil and criminal law.
9. Discuss legal issues relevant to psychiatric/mental health nursing.
10. Differentiate between *malpractice* and *negligence.*
11. Identify behaviors relevant to the psychiatric/mental health setting for which specific malpractice action could be taken.

KEY TERMS

assault	libel
autonomy	Kantianism
battery	malpractice
beneficence	moral behavior
bioethics	natural law
Christian ethics	negligence
civil law	nonmaleficence
common law	privileged communication
defamation of character	right
criminal law	slander
ethical dilemma	statutory law
ethical egoism	torts
ethics	utilitarianism
false imprisonment	values
informed consent	values clarification
justice	

CHAPTER OUTLINE/LECTURE NOTES

I.   Introduction
     A. Nurses are constantly faced with the challenge of making difficult decisions regarding good and evil or life

and death.

    B. Legislation determines what is "right" or "good" within a society.

II.   Definitions

    A. Ethics: a branch of philosophy dealing with values related to human conduct, to the rightness and wrongness of certain actions, and to the goodness and badness of the motives and ends of such actions.

    B. Bioethics: applies to ethics when they refer to concepts within the scope of medicine, nursing, and allied health.

    C. Moral behavior: conduct that results from serious critical thinking about how individuals ought to treat others.

    D. Values: personal beliefs about the truth, beauty, or worth of a thought, object, or behavior.

    E. Values clarification: a process of self-discovery by which people identify their personal values and their value rankings.

    F. Right: that to which an individual is entitled (by ethical or moral standards) to have, or to do, or to receive from within the limits of the law.

    G. Absolute right: when there is no restriction whatsoever upon the individual's entitlement.

    H. Legal right: a right upon which the society has agreed and formalized into law.

III.   Ethical Considerations

    A. Theoretical perspectives

        1. Utilitarianism. An ethical theory that promotes action based on the end results that produced the most good (happiness) for the most people.

        2. Kantianism. Suggests that decisions and actions are bound by a sense of duty. Also called deontology.

        3. Christian ethics. Do unto others as you would have them do unto you; and alternatively, do not do unto others what you would not have them do unto you.

        4. Natural law theories. Do good and avoid evil. Evil acts are never condoned, even if they are intended to advance the noblest of ends.

        5. Ethical egoism. Decisions are based on what is best for the individual making the decision.

    B. Ethical dilemmas

        1. Ethical dilemmas occur when moral appeals can be made for taking each of two opposing courses of action.

        2. Taking no action is considered an action taken.

    C. Ethical principles

        1. Autonomy. This principle emphasizes the status of persons as autonomous moral agents whose right to determine their destinies should always be respected.

        2. Beneficence. Refers to one's duty to benefit or promote the good of others.

        3. Nonmaleficence. Abstaining from negative acts toward another, including acting carefully to avoid harm.

        4. Justice. Principle based upon the notion of a hypothetical social contract between free, equal, and rational persons. The concept of justice reflects a duty to treat all individuals equally and fairly.

    D. A model for making ethical decisions

        1. Assessment

        2. Problem identification

        3. Explore the benefits and consequences of each alternative

        4. Consider principles of ethical theories

        5. Select an alternative

        6. Act upon the decision made and communicate decision to others

        7. Evaluate outcomes

    E. Ethical decision making -- a case study

    F. Ethical issues in psychiatric/mental health nursing

        1. The right to refuse medication

        2. The right to the least restrictive treatment alternative

IV.   Legal Considerations

    A. Nurse practice acts - defines the legal parameters of professional and practical nursing.

    B. Type of law

        1. Statutory law - those that have been enacted by legislative bodies, such as a county or city council, state legislature, or the Congress of the United States.

        2. Common law - derived from decisions made in previous cases.

    C. Classification within statutory and common law

        1. Civil law - protects the private and property rights of individuals and businesses.

           a. Torts - a violation of a civil law in which an individual has been wronged. Torts may be intentional

or nonintentional.
      b. Contracts - compensation or performance of the obligation set forth in the contract is sought.
    2. Criminal law - provides protection from conduct deemed injurious to the public welfare.
  D. Legal issues in psychiatric/mental health nursing
    1. Confidentiality and right to privacy
      a. Doctrine of privileged communication
    2. Informed consent
    3. Restraints and seclusion
      a. False imprisonment
    4. Commitment issues
      a. Voluntary admission
      b. Involuntary commitment
      c. Emergency commitments
      d. The "mentally ill" patient in need of treatment
      e. The gravely disabled patient
  E. Nursing liability
    1. Malpractice and negligence
    2. Types of lawsuits that occur in psychiatric nursing
      a. Breach of confidentiality
      b. Defamation of character
        (1) Libel
        (2) Slander
      c. Invasion of privacy
      d. Assault and battery
      e. False imprisonment
  F. Avoiding liability
    1. Practice within the scope of the nurse practice set.
    2. Observe the hospital's and department's policy manuals.
    3. Measure up to established practice standards.
    4. Always put the patient's rights and welfare first.
    5. Develop and maintain a good interpersonal relationship with each patient and his or her family.
V.   Summary
VI.   Review Questions

LEARNING ACTIVITY

ETHICAL AND LEGAL ISSUES IN PSYCHIATRIC/MENTAL HEALTH NURSING

Identify the following key terms associated with ethical and legal issues in psychiatric/mental health nursing with the descriptions/definitions listed below.

a. assault
b. battery
c. beneficence
d. Christian ethics
e. torts
f. common law
g. libel
h. ethical egoism
i. false imprisonment

j. Kantianism
k. malpractice
l. natural law
m. nonmaleficence
n. slander
o. statutory law
p. utilitarianism
q. civil law
r. criminal law

_____ 1. Ethical theory by which decisions are based on a sense of duty.

_____ 2. Writing false and malicious information about a person.

_____ 3. The unconsented touching of another person.

_____ 4. Provides protection from conduct deemed injurious to the public welfare.

_____ 5. Abstaining from negative acts toward another, including acting carefully to avoid harm.

_____ 6. An act that results in a person's genuine fear and apprehension that he or she will be touched without consent.

_____ 7. The ethical theory in which evil acts are never condoned, even if they are intended to advance the noblest of ends.

_____ 8. A violation of a civil law in which an individual has been wronged.

_____ 9. The ethical theory based on that which ensures the greatest happiness to the greatest number of people.

_____ 10. The deliberate and unauthorized confinement of a person within fixed limits by the use of threat or force.

_____ 11. The failure of a professional to perform or to refrain from performing in a manner expected from a reputable member within the profession.

_____ 12. An ethical principle that refers to one's duty to benefit or promote the good of others.

_____ 13. Law that has been enacted by legislative bodies.

_____ 14. Verbalizing false and malicious information about a person.

_____ 15. An ethical theory that espouses making decisions based on what is most advantageous for the person making the decision.

_____ 16. Law that is derived from decisions made in previous cases.

_____ 17. Law that protects the private and property rights of individuals and businesses.

_____ 18. The ethical theory that espouses "Do unto others as you would have others do unto you."

ETHICAL THEORIES

Utilitarianism

Kantianism (Deontology)

Christian Ethics

Natural Law Theories

Ethical Egoism

ISSUES IN PSYCHIATRIC/ MENTAL HEALTH NURSING

ETHICAL ISSUES

a. The Right to Refuse Medication
b. The Right to the Least Restrictive Treatment Alternative

LEGAL ISSUES

a. Confidentiality and Right to Privacy
b. Informed Consent
c. Restraints and Seclusion
d. Commitment Issues

TYPES OF LAWSUITS THAT OCCUR IN PSYCHIATRIC NURSING

BREACH OF CONFIDENTIALITY

DEFAMATION OF CHARACTER
   a. Libel
   b. Slander

INVASION OF PRIVACY

ASSAULT AND BATTERY

FALSE IMPRISONMENT

APPENDIX: ANSWERS TO LEARNING ACTIVITIES

CHAPTER 1

Exercise 1. Hormonal response to stress.

1. c
2. e
3. a
4. d
5. b

Exercise 2. Holmes and Rahe Social Readjustment Rating Scale

Each student self-administers the evaluation form to determine risk of physical illness due to stress. Method of scoring is included at the bottom of the form.

Exercise 3. Case Study

A. Precipitating Factors:

    1. Genetic influences:
       a. Father and brother both alcoholics
       b. Mother, heavy smoker, died of lung cancer

    2. Past experiences:
       a. First drink at age 12
       b. Increased amount and frequency since that time
       c. Hospitalized three months ago. Diagnosis: ulcer
       d. Erratic work history related to drinking
       e. Fired from his most recent job yesterday

    3. Existing conditions:
       a. Smokes three packages of cigarettes per day
       b. Severe financial difficulties
       c. Supportive wife
       d. No insight into his drinking behavior (blames his boss each time he is fired)

B. Precipitating Stressor: drank two fifths of bourbon

CHAPTER 2

Exercise 1. Please see Figure 2.3 in the text for an explanation of this activity.

Exercise 2. Ego Defense Mechanisms - Definitions

Exercise 3. The Grief Response

1. Anger
2. Denial
3. Acceptance
4. Bargaining
5. Depression
6. Anger
7. Denial
8. Depression
9. Bargaining
10. Acceptance

CHAPTER 3

Exercise 1. Three Components of the Personality

1. id
2. superego
3. ego
4. id
5. id
6. ego
7. superego
8. id
9. ego
10. superego

Exercise 2. Erikson's Stages of Development

1. e
2. b
3. l
4. h
5. o
6. d
7. g

8. n
9. i
10. f
11. j
12. a
13. p
14. k
15. c
16. m

Exercise 3. Stages of Moral Development

1. b
2. f
3. e
4. c
4. a
6. d

CHAPTER 4

Exercise 1. Essential Conditions for Therapeutic Relationship Development

1. b
2. d
3. a
4. c
5. e

Exercise 2. Phases of Relationship Development

1. b
2. a
3. c
4. b
5. d
6. a
7. c
8. d
9. d
10. c

CHAPTER 5

Exercise: Interpersonal Communication Techniques

1. Voicing doubt (T)
2. Belittling feelings (N)
3. Focusing (T)
4. Giving recognition (T)
5. Indicating an external source of power (N)
6. Reflecting (T)
7. Defending (N)
8. Exploring (T)
9. Verbalizing the implied (T)

10.	Giving reassurance (N)
11.	Restating (T)
12.	Giving advice (N)
13.	Giving broad openings (T)
14.	Rejecting (N)
15.	Requesting an explanation (N)

CHAPTER 6

Exercise: Case Study

1.	Assessment data
	a.	Picks up a chair, as if to use it for protection. Threatened to harm anyone who came close to him in the department store.
	b.	Talks and laughs to himself, and tilts his head to the side.
	c.	Keeps to himself, and walks away when anyone approaches him.
	d.	Appearance is unkempt. Clothes are dirty and wrinkled, hair is oily and uncombed, and there is obvious body odor about him.

2.	Nursing diagnoses
	a.	High risk for violence: directed toward others
	b.	Sensory-perceptual alteration (hallucinations)
	c.	Social isolation
	d.	Self-care deficit

3.	Outcome criteria
	a.	Sam has not harmed self or others.
	b.	Sam is able to define and test reality.
	c.	Sam approaches others in an appropriate manner for 1:1 interaction. Attends group activities voluntarily.
	d.	Sam carries out personal care independently and willingly.

4.	Some appropriate nursing interventions include:
	a.	Remove dangerous objects from patient's environment.
	b.	Redirect violent behavior with physical outlets.
	c.	Have sufficient staff available to indicate show of strength.
	d.	Administer antipsychotic medication, as ordered (scheduled and prn)
	e.	Encourage patient to share content of hallucination
	f.	Attend groups with patient until he feels comfortable attending alone
	g.	Give positive feedback for voluntary interactions with others
	h.	Encourage patient to be as independent with self-care activities as possible
	i.	Give positive feedback for self-care activities performed independently

CHAPTER 7

Exercise 1. Family Genogram

Have students refer to Figure 7.1 in the text to construct their own genogram.

Exercise 2. Group Attendance

Students should prepare a written report of their attendance in a group describing:
a.	type of group attended
b.	type of leadership identified
c.	member roles identified

d.   description of group dynamics

CHAPTER 8

Exercise 1. The Interdisciplinary Team

1.   recreational therapist
2.   art therapist
3.   clinical psychologist
4.   chaplain
5.   dietitian
6.   music therapist
7.   clinical nurse specialist
8.   psychiatrist
9.   staff nurse
10.   social worker
11.   occupational therapist

Exercise 2. Basic Assumptions of Milieu Therapy

1.   e
2.   a
3.   g
4.   f
5.   b
6.   d
7.   c

CHAPTER 9

Exercise 1. Types of Crises

1.   f
2.   b
3.   a
4.   e
5.   d
6.   c

Exercise 2. Problem-solving a Crisis

1.   Unresolved separation-individuation tasks
      Unmet dependency needs
      Dysfunctional grieving

2.   To develop a realistic and positive self-perception independent from parents.
      Relinquishing need to secure personal identity through interaction with others.
      To progress through the grief process triggered by loss of previous lifestyle and come to terms with acceptance of the change.

3.   Explore with Jane those aspects which cannot be changed. For example:
      a.   Ted's job requires that he live in the new town.
      b.   Jane's family will continue to live in the town from which they moved.

4.   Alternatives include:

       a.   Stay with Ted and accept the move (an alternative that is developmentally appropriate for Jane, and that the nurse should encourage).

       b.   Leave Ted and move back to home town where relatives live (a decision based on developmental regression).

5.   Jane will need to weigh the personal benefits and consequences of staying with Ted in the new town and working to accept the move, or leaving him and moving back to live near her relatives.

6.   Once Jane has made a decision, she may need assistance from the nurse to help her accept it and adapt to the change. Either decision will undoubtedly trigger a grief response, and assistance in progression to acceptance may be required. Jane must make the decision independently, based on knowledge and understanding of what each would mean for her. A decision to remain with Ted will require work on Jane's part to separate adaptively from her parents and form an independent identity (tasks which have gone unfulfilled by Jane). New coping strategies will have to be developed.

CHAPTER 10

Exercise 1. Inventory of vulnerability to stress

Each student self-administers and scores own evaluation. Explanation of the score is included.

Exercise 2. Stress diary.

Each student keeps a record of adaptation to stress. Group discussion is encouraged.

CHAPTER 11

Exercise: Assertive Techniques

    1.   d
    2.   f
    3.   j
    4.   h
    5.   a
    6.   c
    7.   e
    8.   i
    9.   g
  10.   b

CHAPTER 12

Exercise: Psychotropic Medication Quiz

1.   increase levels of norepinephrine and serotonin
2.   sudden lifts in mood (may indicate suicidal intention)
3.   depending upon the medication, from 1 to 4 weeks
4.   a.   amitriptyline (Elavil)
        b.   phenelzine (Nardil)
5.   a.   dry mouth (offer sugarless candy, ice, frequent sips of water)
        b.   constipation (increase fluids and foods high in fiber)
        c.   sedation (request physician to order given at bedtime)
        d.   orthostatic hypotension (teach patient to rise slowly from a sitting or lying position; take vital signs

every shift)

     e.   lowers seizure threshold (closely observe patient, especially those with history of seizures)

6.   Hypertensive crisis: nurse should be on the alert for symptoms of severe occipital headache, palpitations, nausea and vomiting, nuchal rigidity, fever, sweating, marked increase in blood pressure, chest pain, coma. Patient must avoid foods high in tyramine, such as aged cheeses, pickled herring, preserved meats, beer, wine, chocolate, sour cream, yogurt, over-the-counter cold medications, diet pills.

7.   Mania. Lithium has a lag time of 1 to 3 weeks. Antipsychotics are prescribed to decrease the hyperactivity on an immediate basis until the lithium can take effect.

8.   Therapeutic range: 0.6 to 1.5 mEq/L. Initial signs and symptoms of lithium toxicity are blurred vision, ataxia, tinnitus, persistent nausea and vomiting, severe diarrhea.

9.   a.   Give with food.
    b.   Ensure patient gets adequate sodium in diet.
    c.   Ensure patient drinks 2500 to 3000 cc fluid per day.
    d.   Check for lithium levels before administering dose.
    e.   Monitor patient's intake and output.
    f.   May need to instruct patient on diet to prevent weight gain.

10.   CNS depression

11.   Benzodiazepines: chlordiazepoxide (Librium) and diazepam (Valium)

12.   drowsiness, sedation, confusion, orthostatic hypotension

13.   patient must be instructed not to stop taking the drugs abruptly

14.   decreases levels or activity of dopamine

15.   chlorpromazine (Thorazine) and fluphenazine (Prolixin)

16.   decreased libido; retrograde ejaculation; gynecomastia; amenorrhea; weight gain

17.   sore throat, fever, malaise

18.   severe muscle rigidity, fever up to 107 degrees F, tachycardia, tachypnea, fluctuations in blood pressure, diaphoresis, and rapid deterioration of mental status to stupor and coma

19.   a.   pseudoparkinsonism (tremor, shuffling gait, drooling, rigidity)
    b.   akinesia (muscular weakness)
    c.   akathisia (continuous restlessness and fidgeting)
    d.   dystonia (spasms of face, arms, legs, and neck)
    e.   oculogyric crisis (uncontrolled rolling back of the eyes)
    f.   sometimes tardive dyskinesia is considered as an extrapyramidal system (bizarre facial and tongue movements, stiff neck, and difficulty swallowing)

20   antiparkinsonian agents: benztropine (Cogentin) and trihexyphenidyl (Artane)

CHAPTER 13

Exercise: Electroconvulsive Therapy

    1.   c
    2.   j
    3.   f
    4.   b
    5.   h
    6.   a
    7.   d
    8.   i
    9.   g
    10.   e

CHAPTER 14

Exercise: Techniques for Modifying Patient Behavior

    1.   c

2. i
3. f
4. b
5. j
6. e
7. g
8. k
9. a
10. h
11. l
12. d

CHAPTER 15

Exercise: Disorders of Infancy, Childhood, or Adolescence

1. c
2. h
3. l
4. b
5. k
6. d
7. j
8. f
9. m
10. a
11. g
12. i
13. e

CHAPTER 16

Exercise: Organic Mental Disorders

1. C; I
2. C; I
3. A; R
4. A; R
5. A; R
6. C; I
7. C; I
8. A; R
9. A; R
10. A; R

CHAPTER 17

Exercise: Symptoms Associated with Psychoactive Substances

Drugs	Use	Intoxication	Withdrawal
CNS Depressants Examples: Alcohol Anxiolytics Sedatives Hypnotics	Relaxation, loss of inhibitions, lack of concentration, drowsiness, slurred speech	Aggressiveness, disinhibition, impaired judgment, incoordination, unsteady gait, slurred speech, disorientation, confusion	Tremors, nausea/ vomiting, insomnia, seizures, hallucinations, irritability
CNS Stimulants Examples: Amphetamines Caffeine Cocaine Nicotine	Hyperactivity, agitation, euphoria, insomnia, anorexia, increased pulse	Euphoria, grandiosity, fighting, elevated vital signs, nausea and vomiting, psychomotor agitation	Anxiety, depressed mood, insomnia or hypersomnia, craving for the drug, suicidal ideas (with amphetamines and cocaine)
Opioids Examples: Opium Morphine Codeine Heroin Meperidine	Euphoria, lethargy, drowsiness, lack of motivation	Euphoria, lethargy, somnolence, apathy, dysphoria, impaired judgment, slurred speech, constipation, decreased respiratory rate and blood pressure	Craving for the drug, nausea/vomiting, muscle aches, lacrimation, rhinorrhea, piloerection or sweating, diarrhea, yawning, fever, insomnia
Hallucinogens Examples: Mescaline LSD PCP	Visual hallucinations, disorientation, confusion, paranoia, euphoria, anxiety, panic, increased pulse	Belligerence, impulsiveness, psychomotor agitation, increased heart rate and blood pressure, ataxia, seizures, panic reaction, delirium	The occurrence of a withdrawal syndrome with these substances has not been established.
Cannabis Examples: Marijuana Hashish	Relaxation, talkativeness, lowered inhibitions, euphoria, mood swings	Impaired judgment, loss of recent memory, tremors, muscle rigidity, conjunctival redness, panic, paranoia	If high doses are used for a prolonged period, symptoms of nervousness, tremor, insomnia and restlessness may occur upon cessation of use.

CHAPTER 18

Exercise 1. Behaviors Associated with Schizophrenia

1. g
2. d
3. o

4.   n
5.   m
6.   a
7.   h
8.   k
9.   b
10.   i
11.   c
12.   j
13.   e
14.   l
15.   f

Exercise 2. Symptoms of Schizophrenia

1.   paranoia
2.   delusion of grandeur
3.   echolalia
4.   imitation
5.   nihilistic delusion
6.   anhedonia
7.   body rocking
8.   regression
9.   anergia
10.   apathy
11.   delusion of reference

CHAPTER 19

Exercise 1. Symptoms of Mood Disorders

1.   c
2.   f
3.   a
4.   d
5.   b
6.   b
7.   e
8.   a
9.   e
10.   a
11.   b
12.   e
13.   f

Exercise 2. Facts and Fables About Suicide

1.   F
2.   T
3.   T
4.   F
5.   F
6.   F
7.   T
8.   T
9.   F

10.   F

CHAPTER 20

Exercises: Behaviors Associated with Anxiety Disorders

   1.   c
   2.   g
   3.   b
   4.   d
   5.   f
   6.   a
   7.   c
   8.   e
   9.   d
10.   f
11.   b
12.   c
13.   g
14.   e
15.   d

CHAPTER 21

Exercise: Behaviors Associated with Somatoform Disorders

1.   b; Chronic pain
2.   e; Body image disturbance
3.   d; Sensory-perceptual alteration
4.   a; Ineffective individual coping
5.   c; Fear

CHAPTER 22

Exercise: Behaviors Associated with Dissociative Disorders

1.   c
2.   e
3.   a
4.   g
5.   b
6.   f
7.   d

CHAPTER 23

Values clarification. Students provide their own answers.

CHAPTER 24

Exercise: Case Study

1. 30 years old
   never married
   successful
   active social life/many friends
   no significant other at this time
   recent mastectomy for malignancy
   physical condition good
   sad, tired
   trouble sleeping and concentrating
   unable to work
   personal statement of dissatisfaction with appearance
   personal statement of "My personal life is over."

2. a. Dysfunctional grieving related to loss of right breast evidenced by sadness, fatigue, difficulty sleeping and concentrating, inability to work.

   b. Impaired adjustment related to loss of right breast evidenced by, "No man will ever want to have anything to do with me because of the way I look. My personal life is over."

3. See Table 24.2 "Care Plan for the Patient with Adjustment Disorder."

4. The patient:
   a. is able to verbalize acceptable behaviors associated with each stage of the grief process.
   b. demonstrates a reinvestment in the environment.
   c. is able to accomplish activities of daily living independently.
   d. demonstrates ability for adequate occupational and social functioning.
   e. verbalizes awareness of change in body image and effect it will have on her life style.
   f. is able to problem solve and set realistic goals for the future.
   g. demonstrates ability to cope effectively with change in body image.

CHAPTER 25

Exercise: Psychological Factors Affecting Physical Condition

1. d
2. c
3. a
4. b
5. c
6. a
7. a
8. a
9. b
10. d

CHAPTER 26

Exercise: Personality Disorders

  1. d
  2. j
  3. f
  4. a
  5. e
  6. i
  7. c
  8. h
  9. g
10. k
11. b

CHAPTER 27

Exercise: Case Study

1. 77 years old
a widow for 20 years
lives alone on small farm
has always been very independent
has become forgetful in last few years
starting to wander
has caring support system in son and daughter

2. a. High risk for trauma related to confusion, disorientation, and wandering.
     b. Altered thought processes related to age-related changes that result in cerebral anoxia evidenced by memory loss, confusion, disorientation, and wandering.

3. See Table 27.2, "Care Plan for the Elderly Patient."

4. The patient:
     a. has not experienced injury.
     b. maintains reality orientation consistent with cognitive level of functioning.
     c. can distinguish between reality- and nonreality-based thinking.

Caregivers and patient:
a. verbalize understanding of possible need for long-term care placement.

CHAPTER 28

Exercise: Acquired Immune Deficiency Syndrome

  1. i
  2. m
  3. e
  4. f
  5. l
  6. c
  7. g
  8. d

9. b
10. k
11. j
12. a
13. h

CHAPTER 29

Exercise: Victims of Violence

1. d
2. i
3. h
4. c
5. g
6. j
7. k
8. a
9. 1
10. f
11. e
12. b

CHAPTER 30

Exercise: Ethical and Legal Issues in Psychiatric/Mental Health Nursing

1. j
2. g
3. b
4. r
5. m
6. a
7. l
8. e
9. p
10. i
11. k
12. c
13. o
14. n
15. h
16. f
17. q
18. d